the touch of healing

the touch of healing

of healing

energizing body, mind, and
spirit with the art of Jin Shin Jyutsu®

Alice Burmeister with Tom Monte

Foreword by Mary Burmeister

Bantam Books
NEW YORK   TORONTO   LONDON   SYDNEY   AUCKLAND

THE TOUCH OF HEALING

A Bantam Book / September 1997

Jin Shin Jyutsu is a registered trademark.

BOOK DESIGN BY VERTIGO DESIGN

Library of Congress Cataloging-in-Publication Data
Burmeister, Alice.
    The touch of healing : energizing body, mind, and spirit with the art
of Jin Shin Jyutsu / Alice Burmeister, with Tom Monte.
        p.   cm.
    Includes bibliographical references (p.) and index.
    ISBN 0-553-37784-1 (pbk.)
    1. Acupressure.   I. Monte, Tom.   II. Title.
RM723.A27B87   1997
615.8′22—DC21   96-36960

Published simultaneously in the United States and Canada

Bantam Books are published by Bantam Books, a division of Bantam Doubleday Dell Publishing Group, Inc. Its trademark, consisting of the words "Bantam Books" and the portrayal of a rooster, is Registered in U.S. Patent and Trademark Office and in other countries. Marca Registrada. Bantam Books, 1540 Broadway, New York, New York 10036.

PRINTED IN THE UNITED STATES OF AMERICA
20 19 18 17 16

IN LOVING MEMORY OF
Gilbert C. Burmeister

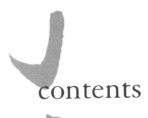

contents

acknowledgments ix

foreword by Mary Burmeister xi

introduction: a simple way for health and balance 1

chapter one
the foundations of the art   11

chapter two
the depths and attitudes 23

chapter three
the trinity flows 43

chapter four
safety energy locks: 1–15 55

chapter five
safety energy locks: 16–26 81

chapter six
the organ flows 97

chapter seven
general daily sequences 133

chapter eight
harmonizing with the fingers and toes 145

chapter nine
first aid and on-the-spot healing 161

appendix 171

bibliography 175

index 177

acknowledgments

THE AUTHORS WISH TO THANK THE FOLLOWING PEOPLE FOR THEIR HELP AND ADVICE: Mary Burmeister, David Burmeister, Pat Meador, Muriel Carlton, Philomena Dooley, Wayne Hackett, Susan Brooks, Lynne Pflueger, Waltraud Riegger-Krause, Mathias Roth, Jed Schwartz, Dr. Haruki Kato, Sara Harper, Janet Oliver, Priscilla Pitman, Phyllis Singer, Brian Tart, Doyle Darragh, Jean Fraschina, Jeanette Chorlian, Norm Goldstein, Ian Kraut, Karen Moore, Steve Black, Connie Fisher, David Reynolds, Reuben and Rhoda Draisin, and all the Jin Shin Jyutsu students and clients whose numerous stories appear throughout this book.

foreword

My parents were storytellers. I grew up hearing stories from mythology and ancient times. I am often reminded of one that occurred in a marketplace in ancient Greece.

A FIGHT BROKE out between two men. Among the bystanders was Pythagoras, the great mathematician and philosopher. Just as one of the combatants was about to strike the other with his sword, Pythagoras picked up his lute and plucked a single, clear note. Upon hearing this sound, the angry man lay down his sword and walked away.

Pythagoras' understanding of harmonic relationships helped him choose the one perfect tone that could pacify the man.

Jin Shin Jyutsu helps us find that tone, the perfect expression of harmony, that exists within everyone. It is a philosophy, a psychology, and a physiology. It demonstrates a way of Being to understand cosmic oneness and to know and help ourselves.

A friend once remarked that Jin Shin Jyutsu is "complicatedly simple." One who understands and sincerely respects the profound significance of this Physio-Philosophy and follows its procedures accordingly should be neither intimidated by its magnitude nor apprehensive about practicing it. It is not application of technique; it is demonstration of art, simply Being the channel through which flow the infinite aesthetic powers of the Creator.

Jin Shin Jyutsu is a lifelong journey toward self-knowledge and harmony. This book is a road map for that journey. It will start you in the right direction and show you how to proceed along the way. Learning the route is just the first step. Continuing on the journey depends on complying with the art's established procedures and on unencumbered communion with the Creator.

May your journey be as blessed as my own.

Mary Burmeister

the touch of healing

introduction

a simple way for health and balance

In 1977 Celeste Martin attended a real estate convention in New Orleans—a rare event for her, since she traveled only when her health would permit it. Celeste suffered from phlebitis, a life-threatening disorder that causes blood clots. As a preventive measure, she was taking daily doses of a blood-thinning medication as well as having her blood regularly monitored by physicians.

Celeste had suffered from the disease for nineteen years and had been frequently hospitalized for it. The large saphenous veins in both her legs had been removed due to the clots. In addition, two clots had formed in her lungs. These pulmonary embolisms could have been fatal without proper medical intervention. Smaller embolisms were causing her to have numerous transient ischemic attacks, or ministrokes. Chronic swelling and pain from poor circulation forced her to wear elastic bandages around her legs.

Now, in a kind of rebellion against the limitations that her disease imposed, Celeste decided to get away for a week. At the convention, quite out of the blue, a man by the name of Charles approached her and offered her some strange advice: "If you don't want to continue looking like you're half dead, I know a woman who can help you."

The woman to whom Charles was referring was Mary Burmeister, a teacher and practitioner of a little-known healing art called Jin Shin Jyutsu. When Charles explained that Jin Shin Jyutsu could achieve powerful results using nothing more than a simple application of the hands, Celeste was immediately skeptical. Having worked as a nurse for twenty-one years, her training and experience had given her no intellectual framework in which to place such information. She returned home to New Jersey feeling that Charles was an interesting man but of no real relevance to her.

A month later Celeste came home from work with a strange tingling feeling around her face, as if she had walked into a thick spiderweb. Later that day she lost all feeling and strength in the left side of her body. Remarkably, Charles called that very night to see how she was doing. When she told him her symptoms, he told her to hang up and stay by the phone; he would call her right back. Charles phoned Mary Burmeister, who instructed him on how Celeste could help relieve her symptoms. Charles called back and conveyed the information to Celeste. For the next couple of hours, her children followed the instructions. They placed their hands upon the appropriate areas of their mother's body. By two o'clock that morning, her symptoms were gone.

"I would have been hospitalized the next day," recalls Celeste, "but instead I went to work." Charles phoned later that day. When she told him the symptoms were gone, he replied, "Now will you believe what I told you?"

Celeste did believe him, and in early April she went to Scottsdale, Arizona, for ten days to receive Jin Shin Jyutsu. Mary Burmeister was out of town at the time, so longtime Jin Shin practitioner Pat Meader performed the art on Celeste. Pat gave Celeste two sessions a day, one in the morning and the other in the afternoon. During her ninth session Celeste had a strange experience of being transformed, as if some deep blockage inside of her were releasing. She felt as if energy were flowing freely inside of her. Later that day Celeste received a telephone call. Without thinking, she got up from the place where she had been sitting and walked to the phone—only to realize, after she picked up the phone, that she felt no pain in her legs. Quite the opposite—her legs felt strong and nimble. Suddenly, she let out a shout of joy—"I have no pain in my legs!"

Upon her return to New Jersey, Celeste was met by her cousin at the airport. Her cousin hardly recognized her. Once she was home, Celeste underwent a full medical examination, which showed that her blood pressure and blood-clotting mechanisms were all normal. "What have you been doing?" her doctor asked. Celeste explained. "Well, whatever it is, keep doing it."

At that point Celeste knew she was all right. "I had no more fear," she said. "I had always been living in fear that a clot would get loose and kill me suddenly. Now all that fear was gone." At 44 years of age, she felt as if she were reborn.

Celeste's story is remarkable, but it is by no means atypical. The lives of countless other people have been dramatically improved after an exposure to Jin Shin Jyutsu. Like Celeste, many of them were initially skeptical about its ability to help them. The art is so disarmingly simple and gentle that many wonder as to its potency. Yet its subtle character is one of the primary components of its effectiveness. Because it is so gentle and noninvasive, Jin Shin Jyutsu allows the recipient to feel more at ease and receptive to the healing process.

Jin Shin Jyutsu is much more than a glorified placebo, however. Its principles and practices are firmly rooted in ancient, long-forgotten healing traditions. It was rediscovered, as we shall shortly see, after years of meticulous, systematic research by one man—

Master Jiro Murai. Murai subsequently passed this knowledge along to Mary Burmeister.

Mary Burmeister's husband, Gil, shares the following story, which serves as an excellent illustration of both the subtlety and the power of this healing art. After World War II Gil had been serving in Japan as a civilian employee of the American military. Soon after Mary arrived in Japan, she met Gil, who began to court her. Meanwhile, Mary was studying with Jiro Murai. At the time Gil was suffering from chronic rectal itching, which eventually developed into a fistula that had to be removed surgically. Yet even after the operation, the itching persisted. No medication could relieve the discomfort. A year after the surgery, Mary suggested that Gil see Jiro Murai. Gil agreed.

Gil entered Master Murai's sparse room—the only visible furnishing was a white mat lying at the center of the clean hardwood floor. Murai invited Gil to lie down on the mat. Gil complied, and the teacher placed his hands upon him. The instant Gil felt Murai's touch, a tremendous wave of energy seemed to penetrate his body. "I had this sensation of rushing energy," Gil recalled many years later. He quickly fell asleep and remained so for a couple of hours. In the meantime Murai did nothing more than move his hands to different parts of Gil's body. When Gil later awoke, the itching was gone. It never returned.

Murai was unquestionably a brilliant man, and his painstaking research gave him a profound understanding of the intricacies of the human body. This understanding enabled him to zero in on the source of Gil's suffering. More importantly, however, it led Murai to recover an awareness of a healing art that is both simple and wide-ranging in its application. Anyone who wished to, he realized, could learn this art and use it for their own benefit and for the benefit of others. In order to provide future generations with the opportunity to learn Jin Shin Jyutsu, he imparted all that he could to the young Mary Burmeister.

Today, more than forty years later, Mary has taught Jin Shin

Jyutsu to students from all over the world. One of them is Celeste Martin. Shortly after she experienced her remarkable recovery, Celeste decided to devote herself to the study and practice of Jin Shin Jyutsu. In fact, it wasn't long after Celeste began to study it that she was able to use it to help someone else—her mother.

In April 1979 Celeste's mother suffered a fall that shattered her hip. The trauma brought on congestive heart failure and sent her into a coma. Celeste called Mary Burmeister to ask if Jin Shin Jyutsu could do anything for her mother. Mary gave her instructions on the appropriate areas to place her hands. The next day Celeste was at her comatose mother's bedside.

"Mary had instructed me as to where I should place my right hand and my left hand," Celeste recalls. "But I didn't know what I was doing. I didn't know what I could do, if anything at all." Nevertheless, Celeste began to perform Jin Shin Jyutsu as Mary had instructed.

Celeste's mother had been catheterized. A plastic bag hung beside her bed, into which had drained about an inch of urine. Celeste had performed about fifteen minutes of Jin Shin Jyutsu when suddenly she looked up and saw that the bag was full, even overflowing. Immediately she rang for a nurse, who hurried into the room. Upon seeing the bag, the nurse said to Celeste, "Well, that's strange. I was just in here a little while ago, and there was little or no drainage in the bag."

As the nurse said those words, Celeste's mother opened her eyes and said, "Is that you, Celeste?" From that moment on, Celeste's mother gradually got stronger. Eventually she made a full recovery.

"I was shocked and amazed," said Celeste. "I was also scared. I didn't know that a simple person like me could do these things. I accepted that that was an ability of Mary's, but now I realized and was humbled by the fact that people could also be helped through me."

Celeste's experience with her mother exemplifies the wonderful accessibility of Jin Shin Jyutsu. With only a minimum of experience, she had been able to assist greatly in her mother's healing process. Each one of us has the same potential. An awareness of Jin Shin Jyutsu's basic concepts and practices provides a wonderful tool for offering help to our loved ones. And as the following story illustrates, it can greatly enhance our ability to help ourselves.

In 1983, at the age of 38, Amy began to experience significant joint pain and inflammation. Occasionally the pain in her knees and feet would become so intense that it prevented her from walking for days at a time. At first her physician thought she suffered from rheumatoid arthritis, but tests failed to confirm the presence of any specific joint disease. Her doctor then prescribed cortisone and anti-inflammatory medication for her condition.

In 1985 tests revealed that Amy's liver had become enlarged. Further tests, including a liver biopsy, ruled out cancer but were unable to provide any clear diagnosis. Meanwhile, her symptoms worsened. In 1988 tests revealed clearly that her liver was dysfunctioning. Her doctors told her that she had connective tissue disease, a nonspecific term for numerous disorders.

Finally, her doctors diagnosed Amy as having lupus, an illness in which the body's immune system attacks connective tissue and essential organs, including the brain and kidneys.

In the summer of 1990, Amy's condition took a dramatic turn for the worse. Tests revealed that her kidney function had been cut to 50 percent of maximum. The kidney specialist who was monitoring Amy informed her that if her kidney function fell to 20 percent or lower, she would need kidney dialysis.

Just when it seemed that things could not get any worse, Amy was involved in a car accident that left her with severe neck pain. Ironically, this accident proved to be her doorway back to health.

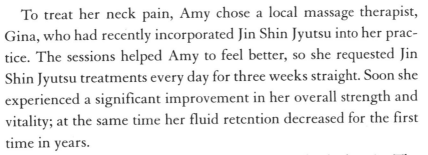

To treat her neck pain, Amy chose a local massage therapist, Gina, who had recently incorporated Jin Shin Jyutsu into her practice. The sessions helped Amy to feel better, so she requested Jin Shin Jyutsu treatments every day for three weeks straight. Soon she experienced a significant improvement in her overall strength and vitality; at the same time her fluid retention decreased for the first time in years.

The following month Amy had her kidneys checked again. The tests showed that their function had fallen to 25 percent. Her physician told her that if her kidney function dropped five more points, he would be forced to refer her to a kidney transplant team.

In April 1994 tests showed that her kidneys were functioning at only 21 percent of maximum—dangerously close to the precipice. Convinced that it was just a matter of time, her doctor advised Amy that in the near future she would have to have a kidney transplant or else undergo regular dialysis.

"After I got the test results, I left my doctor's office and sat in my car, and I thought about my future and what I would do," Amy recalls. "I decided right then that I was not going to have a transplant or dialysis. I didn't know what I was going to do, but I was not going to accept either of those choices."

The next thing she did was telephone Mary's son, David Burmeister, at the Jin Shin Jyutsu office in Scottsdale. David encouraged Amy to continue receiving medical care and recommended Marilyn, a longtime practitioner who worked in Amy's hometown, Dallas.

In May 1994 Amy saw Marilyn for the first time. "I knew during that first treatment with Marilyn that something special was happening to me," recalls Amy. "It seemed as if some weight had been lifted from my body." Soon Amy had so much energy that she didn't know what to do with herself. "One day I felt so alive and filled with energy that I cleaned all the baseboards in my house."

From that May onward, Amy saw Marilyn two to three times each week and Gina once a week. Meanwhile, she had been taught a variety of Jin Shin Jyutsu self-help routines that she could use daily to strengthen her condition. Amy applied them diligently.

It was Amy's commitment to the Jin Shin Jyutsu self-help routines, Gina says, that helped turn her condition around. In August 1994 Amy underwent another kidney test. This time things were dramatically different. The tests showed that her kidney function was up to 30 percent. Her doctor marveled at the improvement. "If you get up to 40 percent," he told her, "I'll learn this Jin Shin Jyutsu myself."

Amy's health continued to improve. In August 1995 another test revealed that her kidney function was at 43 percent. Needless to say, she was ecstatic. Eventually, Amy's enthusiasm led her to attend a Jin Shin Jyutsu class to learn how to use it for her family members. She summarizes her experience by saying, "In May 1994, when it seemed like a kidney transplant or dialysis was inevitable, I told a friend that I believed that I was not going to die, that I was going to have a miracle. In some way I was guided to this practice. If I had not had Jin Shin Jyutsu, I would be on dialysis today, or perhaps even be dead."

As the preceding stories clearly illustrate, Jin Shin Jyutsu can enable ordinary people to help themselves and others in seemingly extraordinary ways. It is our hope, in writing this book, to provide the reader an opportunity to do the same. As such, we have written it more for the general reader than for the serious practitioner. It can, however, be used as a reference by both.

What follows, then, is an overview of the essential concepts and practices of Jin Shin Jyutsu, as they were originally set down by Master Jiro Murai. Up until now, anyone wishing to obtain this information would have had to attend an authorized Jin Shin Jyutsu class or else read Mary Burmeister's writings. For the purpose of communicating these ideas to a general readership, we have at-

tempted to present them in uncomplicated, everyday language. In order to retain the flavor of Mary's original teachings, we have included numerous quotations from her texts and lectures. These generally appear at the beginning of each section.

Lastly, we wish to emphasize that this book is not intended as the definitive, comprehensive work on the subject of Jin Shin Jyutsu. The multifaceted, multilayered nature of this healing art makes such an undertaking well beyond the scope of this book. Anyone wishing to supplement the material covered here is strongly encouraged to attend an authorized Jin Shin Jyutsu class. Those interested may contact the Jin Shin Jyutsu office in Scottsdale for more information. The address and phone number are listed in the Appendix.

For most readers, the basic concepts and exercises that are the focus of this book will be more than sufficient. They will provide you with a wide array of tools to balance and maintain physical, emotional, and mental health. You can use them in conjunction with conventional medicine to help yourself and others facilitate the healing process. Or you may use them preventively, to sustain a sense of harmony and well-being. Ultimately, Jin Shin Jyutsu will restore you to a knowledge of yourself and of your long-dormant innate ability to improve the quality of your life.

the foundations of the art

We live in an age of information. The media are able to broadcast global events within seconds of their occurrence. The Internet links us to specialized data. Increasingly, we hope that scientific and technological advances will grant us a better understanding of ourselves, along with the secrets of well-being.

Our growing reliance upon external information has gradually obscured a

A student seeking to familiarize herself with the Art of Jin Shin Jyutsu attended her first class.

During the lunch break, the student introduced herself to the teacher, Mary Burmeister. She confessed to feeling a bit overwhelmed. "I'm afraid that I don't know anything about Jin Shin Jyutsu."

Mary smiled and said, "You already know everything about it."

simple, innate awareness that all of us have long possessed. Inherent in this awareness are all the tools that we need to genuinely enrich our health and the quality of our lives.

The art of Jin Shin Jyutsu enables us to re-experience this awareness. Moreover, it teaches us how to utilize it for greater physical, mental, and spiritual well-being. No complicated technique or effort is required to apply it. Its seeds have lain dormant within us for virtually thousands of years. In order to revive them, we need only heed Plato's teaching that "learning is remembering."

the life in
all things

In ancient times traditional people saw no distinction between body, mind, and spirit. Consequently, the practices they used to assist the body naturally promoted physical, emotional, and spiritual wholeness. Moreover, people saw their health or "harmony" as dependent upon bringing seemingly disparate elements into balance.

Jin Shin Jyutsu (pronounced *jin shin jitsu*) helps us remember that every one of us possesses the simplest instruments needed to bring about harmonious balance—the breath and hands. It reminds us that these instruments are all that we need to enhance our physical and mental vitality, which in turn help eliminate the causes underlying disease, or "disharmony." Most importantly, it reawakens our awareness of the life energy that permeates the universe. This renewed awareness enables us to send life-giving energy through various locations on the body.

The concept of a life energy that pervades the universe and gives life to all things is unfamiliar to many of us. In much of the Western world, we're likely to view life as nothing more than certain chemical processes that make possible the utilization of energy, metabolism, growth, and reproduction.

This concept, given to us by modern science, focuses on the biological aspects of life. From its point of view, life begins and ends with biology, or with the physical part of life. But practitioners of Jin Shin Jyutsu—and indeed, traditional people everywhere—ask themselves: What powers these chemical interactions? What gives life to our organs and systems? What is the force that brings the body to life?

In seeking the answers to these questions, traditional people learned to look beyond to the underlying energy that vitalizes the physical body. They see life as pervaded by a single living force, manifested in every individual organism—plants, insects, animals, and human beings. The ancient Greeks referred to this energy as *pneuma;* the Hindus call it *prana;* the Chinese know it as *chi* (also *qi*), and the Japanese, *ki.*

The recognition of a life energy that animates all living things is not merely a philosophical belief. It is also a practical approach to life and healing. Indeed, virtually all traditional healing systems— from Ayurvedic to Greek and Chinese—are founded on the principle that in order to heal the body, the person must strengthen and harmonize the flow of life energy within. This principle provides the basis for such arts as acupuncture and acupressure, as well as for the healing herbs and foods of Chinese medicine.

Mary Burmeister, who introduced Jin Shin Jyutsu to the Western world more than forty years ago, illustrates the importance of life energy by using a simple analogy: "What makes a car engine start when you turn on the key? The battery of the car. The battery is the necessary energy source for the various functions of the car. Now, what makes a heart beat? What makes breathing possible? What makes digestion possible? The Battery of Life. An energy source is necessary for the body to function. That source is the battery of life."

Our health or harmony depends upon the free and even distribution of this life energy throughout our body, mind, and spirit. When the stress and strain of daily living disrupts the movement of life energy, our mind, body, and spirit are all affected. Not only do we succumb to worry, fear, anger, sadness, and pretensions, but we increase our tendency to become ill or "out of balance."

Quite simply, Jin Shin Jyutsu is a way to balance the life energy. It shows us how to use simple hands-on sequences to restore emotional equilibrium, relieve pain, and release the causes of both acute and chronic conditions. It can be used safely in conjunction with any other therapy or medication. Furthermore, its benefits are cumulative, so that the more we practice it, the greater is our vitality and self-knowledge.

Jin Shin Jyutsu can be used anywhere and at any time. Its methods are so easy and unobtrusive that you may use them on yourself in a crowded bus or in the middle of a difficult meeting. The only thing people may notice—if they notice anything at all—is a more balanced demeanor, an aura of relaxation, and—upon closer examination—that you are holding one or more of your fingers.

the forgotten art,
recently remembered

The name *Jin Shin Jyutsu* means "The Art of the Creator through the person of compassion." The healing art that those words represent is based upon our own natural, innate ability to harmonize ourselves. For thousands of years, ancient peoples used this awareness to heal both themselves and others. But with successive generations this awareness grew dimmer until it was all but forgotten. In the early part of the twentieth century, a Japanese sage named Jiro Murai recovered Jin Shin Jyutsu—out of necessity.

Jiro Murai was born in Taiseimura (currently Kaga City), in Ishikawa Prefecture, in 1886. He was the second son born to his parents. Jiro's father, like his father and so many of his ancestors, was a medical doctor. Since Japanese custom expected that the eldest son would follow in the profession of his father, Jiro was free to choose his own path. He started out as a breeder of silkworms, but he had a reckless nature and overindulged in food and drink— even to the point of entering eating contests, in which he was awarded cash prizes for consuming huge quantities. By the time he was 26, he was seriously ill. A succession of doctors treated him, but his condition only worsened until he was pronounced incurable and given up for terminally ill. As a last request, he asked his family to carry him on a stretcher to their mountain cabin and to leave him there alone for seven days. He asked that they return for him on the eighth day.

There in the cabin Murai fasted, meditated, and practiced various finger postures. During this time he passed in and out of consciousness. His physical body grew colder. But on the seventh day he felt as if he had been lifted out of a deep freeze and thrown into a blazing furnace. When the intense heat subsided, he experienced a tremendous calm and inner peace. To his great surprise, he was healed. He dropped to his knees, gave thanks, and pledged his life to the study of healing.

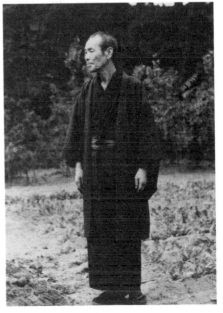

Murai's commitment to understanding the causes of disharmony was profound. Gil Burmeister remembers him as a man obsessed with the pursuit of knowledge: "Jiro did his research among the homeless in Wano Park, in Tokyo. A large population lived in the park. Jiro would take care of the people there and study the incredible variety of illnesses that these people presented. I remember that he went through a period of studying ear problems for a while. He wanted to work on anybody who had any kind of ear complaint. Once he understood ear problems, he'd go on to something else." Murai's prodigious research led him to an awareness of a healing art that he called Jin Shin Jyutsu.

As Murai's understanding of the Art deepened, the meaning of the name *Jin Shin Jyutsu* evolved. At first, he used the words to mean "the Art of Happiness," later "the Art of Longevity." The meaning further evolved to "the Art of Benevolence" and ultimately to "the Art of the Creator through the person of compassion."

Insofar as anyone knows, Jiro Murai never left Japan, but he wanted to make the practice of Jin Shin Jyutsu available to the world. To do that, he selected a young Japanese-American woman named Mary Burmeister.

Born in Seattle, Washington, in 1918, Mary Iino (Mary's maiden name) arrived in Japan in the late 1940s to serve as a translator and to study diplomacy. Highly intelligent and a dedicated student, indeed a natural scholar, Mary had ambitions of entering a Japanese university. In addition, she had the incentive of wanting to overcome the prejudice that was directed against Japanese-Americans in Seattle, and specifically against her family and herself. "I had a chip on my shoulder," she recalls.

Mary knew little of the healing arts when she met Jiro Murai at a mutual friend's house. Murai approached her and offered her a life-altering invitation: "Would you like to study with me to take a gift from Japan to America?" Mary, though taken aback, was strangely open to the suggestion. "Yes" was the only thing she could think to say.

Mary studied with Murai for the next twelve years. Yet shortly after her studies with him began, she fell ill. She was in tremendous pain and weakness and could not get out of bed. Whenever friends came to visit her, they left weeping, uncertain if they would ever see her again.

For more than a month, Murai treated Mary three times each

week, riding the train an hour and a half to her home. Because Mary was so depleted, he would treat her for only five to fifteen minutes at a time. One day after treating her, he told Mary that the next day she would be well. Still weary and in pain, she could hardly believe it. Nevertheless, she awoke the next day without any discomfort and realized that she was completely healed.

Mary later recalled how that illness profoundly shaped her. "Until then I never experienced sickness, never had as much as a headache. In fact, when people had them, I thought to myself, 'cop-out,' that it was a way of avoiding responsibilities." Afterward, she understood that suffering is not feigned. This realization infused her with the compassion necessary to pursue a life devoted to helping others.

For the next forty years, Mary was never again ill. In 1954 she moved back to the United States and settled in Los Angeles, but it wasn't until 1963 that she began to practice Jin Shin Jyutsu actively.

Mary has more than fulfilled Murai's hopes for her. Since the master's death in 1961, she has been the world's foremost teacher of Jin Shin Jyutsu, as well as the embodiment of all that the Art offers. She has tirelessly practiced and taught the Art of Jin Shin Jyutsu throughout the United States and Europe.

Mary describes the essence of Jin Shin Jyutsu with the phrase "TO KNOW (HELP) MY-SELF." As she wrote in one of her texts: "Through Jin Shin Jyutsu our awareness is awakened to the simple fact that all that is needed for harmony and balance with the universe—physically, emotionally, and spiritually— is within myself. Through this awareness, the feeling of complete peace, serenity, security, the oneness within is evident. No person, situation, or thing can take these away from me."

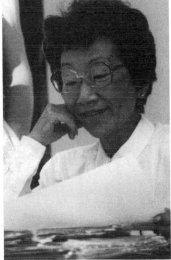

(*PHOTO BY RON THOMPSON*)

the foundation
concepts

By way of introduction, we will now explore the core concepts that form the foundation of Jin Shin Jyutsu. These concepts can be summarized as follows:

- There is a life energy that circulates throughout the universe and within each individual organism.

- This universal life energy manifests itself in varying levels of density. These levels are referred to as *depths*. There are nine depths. At the ninth depth the energy is expressed in its most infinite, undifferentiated form. As it proceeds through each of the successive eight depths, the energy grows denser and gradually encompasses all of the spiritual, psychological, and physical aspects of our existence.

- Breath is the basic expression of the life energy. It enables us to unload accumulated stress and stagnant energy via exhalation. With each inhalation, we receive an abundance of fresh, purified energy.

- When the life energy moves through us without obstruction, we are in perfect harmony. Obstructions—which lead to physical, mental, and emotional disharmony—are created by *attitudes*. There are five basic attitudes: worry, fear, anger, sadness, and pretense (cover-up). All attitudes arise from FEAR, or what Mary refers to as *False Evidence Appearing Real*.

- Life energy moves through the body in distinct pathways, known as *flows*. These flows unify and integrate the body.

- Energy moves down the front of the body and up the back, in a continuous oval. This movement creates a complementary relationship between the upper and lower body as well as the front and the back. Therefore, if the symptom of disharmony appears above the waist, the cause is found below the waist. A similar relationship exists between the back and front of the body.

- There are twenty-six distinct sites, called *safety energy locks,* on each side of the body. These safety energy locks act as circuit-breakers to protect the body when the flow of life energy is blocked. Once a safety energy lock shuts down, it manifests a symptom in the corresponding part of the body. This serves as an alarm that also indicates the source of the imbalance.

- Finally, within each of us an underlying harmony is always present, even when we suffer from some prevailing disharmony or illness. Even though such disharmonies seem to take many different forms, they all arise from the same root cause—blockage of life energy. For this reason, the resultant disharmonies are called *labels.* Big scary labels, such as cancer or heart disease, indicate a lot of blocked or stuck energy. Less fearsome labels, such as simple indigestion or a common cold, arise out of smaller blockages. Any label, regardless of its size, can be helped by freeing up the stagnant energy.

Essential to all of the preceding concepts is the idea of a universal life energy. Jin Shin Jyutsu teaches us that this energy is something more than an abstract, inaccessible force. Moreover, one of the primary ways to facilitate the flow of this energy is actually much more accessible than people think—it is implicit in our every breath.

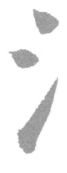

the first gateway
to harmony

We come into the

world with an

exhalation, to clear

and empty us, so that

we can receive. We

never "take" a

breath. We "receive"

a breath.

The first tool for relaxing the body and removing blockages in the life energy is the breath. All we need at any moment is to exhale deeply and allow the new breath to enter our being naturally. With every exhalation, we release piled-up stresses, physical tension, and FEAR. Deep exhalation empties us, so that we can receive more fully the next inhalation and its life-giving energy. Now the life energy can move more fluidly through our system. We can be refreshed and enlivened by the breath—"the purified essence of life."

If you exhale now, you can feel the tension drain from your shoulders, torso, and pelvis—all the way down to your toes. With each breath, you become more relaxed, returning deeper into the harmony, as the tension releases from your body. Receive each breath with awareness and gratitude.

Breath is the basis for energy. The life energy that surrounds us and permeates the universe is always available to us in the form of breath. There is no scarcity of the life energy—it is the most available of all natural resources. So we always have available the power to transform our lives and our world. The key to that transformation is simply to exhale and allow the life energy to fully infuse our being. As Mary says, "In the breath that I am, I am always new."

Mary recalls a man who attended one of her seminars. When it was finished, he dismissed all that she had said. Shortly afterward the man went on a guided tour of the Grand Canyon. When the group got down to the bottom of the canyon, the man became ill and could not go another step. The guide was adamant: "There is no paramedic here, no mule, and no one to carry you out," he said. "You've got to make it on your own." Unfortunately, the man couldn't move. The guide took the group back to the top of the canyon so he could send for help. As the man lay waiting in exhaustion and despair, he remembered Mary's words: *The breath is the ultimate tool. Go into the breath. Exhale and accept the gift that the universe is giving you with every inhalation.* He began to do just that, exhaling and breathing more naturally and rhythmically, receiving life energy with every inhalation. Miraculously, he began to feel stronger. "Pretty soon, he had caught up to his group and made it all the way to the top without any assistance," Mary recalls. Later, the man called Mary to thank her for what she had taught him.

The breath is the simplest and most perfect of all the tools we have at our convenience. It can be used at any waking moment to enhance and balance the life energy, so that we can enter the realm from which harmony and healing flow.

the thirty-six breaths

Here is a simple breathing practice that restores balance to all of the functions within you:

Begin by counting your exhalations. ("One, exhale, inhale. Two, exhale, inhale. Three, exhale, inhale." And so on.) Count until you have completed thirty-six breaths. If you lose count, you can start again. This can be done at one time or throughout the day, counting in four groups of nine. Allow your breathing to unfold naturally. In time, your breathing will automatically become deeper and more rhythmic.

the depths and attitudes

the hands as jumper cables

Throughout the past four decades, Mary Burmeister has seen an average of ten people per day, six days per week. Each session normally lasts an hour. Although many people travel great distances to receive healing from her, she does not see herself as the source of the healing energy. Rather, she believes that every one of us

I don't do anything. The Universal Energy does everything. Therefore, I can take credit for nothing. At the same time, because I do nothing, I never get tired. In all the years that I have jumper-cabled people with contagious diseases, I have never gotten sick from someone else's disease.

—MARY BURMEISTER

23

has the same ability to channel the universal life energy through the body by using our hands. Simply placing one's hands upon the appropriate area allows the life energy to travel through to another part of our own body or to another human being. The universal life energy will penetrate clothing, a cast, a bandage, or a brace. None of these can obstruct the flow of life energy from the practitioner's hands to the recipient.

Visualize the hands as jumper cables. Just apply—no strength is required. There is no need to rub or massage. When she is discussing the application of the jumper cables, Mary reminds her students that Jin Shin Jyutsu is not a technique but an Art. A technique often requires the memorization of specialized rules and a precise "mechanical" application. An art, on the other hand, calls for a breadth of understanding and a flexible, creative approach. Accordingly, there is no absolute way for applying your own jumper cables. Whatever feels the most natural is the right way.

Here are some key points to keep in mind whenever you are jumper-cabling yourself or someone else.

- Relax. If you are unable to relax, just be as you are. There is no need to try to relax. In time you will be able to relax without trying.

- You may sit, stand, or lie down—whatever is most comfortable, convenient, and practical for you.

- Simply apply your hands for a few minutes at a time to each step, or until you can feel an even, rhythmic pulsation.

- Jumper-cabling can be done at any time of day. It is the daily application of the simple sequences that will accomplish results.

The act of jumper-cabling is, in fact, effortlessly simple—we can achieve powerful results merely by holding one of our fingers. As we shall see shortly, each of our fingers is responsible for harmonizing a particular dimension or *depth* of our being. Harmonizing each of these depths enables us to unload those pernicious attitudes (such as fear or sadness) that are the primary causes of stagnant energy and disharmony.

depths and attitudes

Matter is the lowest

level of spirit, and

spirit is the highest

degree of matter.

The vast scope of Jin Shin Jyutsu is most evident in the concept of *depths*. The depths are a practical healing tool as well as a means of understanding how we came into being and how we remain unified with the source of all life.

The depths can be understood as dimensions of being, each one responsible for a specific set of functions within the body, mind, and spirit. All of these dimensions interact with each other and are interdependent. At the same time, each dimension also provides a direct foundation for the next. Thus they reveal the implicit order in life and give us insight into the intention behind each dimension of our being.

The depths also describe the process by which energy becomes form, spirit becomes matter, and each step in creation is built upon the preceding step. Although we define each depth as a stage of creation, it must be remembered that we are never separated from any stage, so that even the most diffuse forms of pure energy are still unified with the physical body itself. Each depth interacts with the others to sustain and integrate the human experience. In short, the interrelatedness of the depths reveals the link between nonphysical and physical reality, between thought and substance, and between the universe and the individual.

Let's pause for a minute and imagine ourselves as originating from an infinite source of energy. This, in fact, is precisely the way that modern science theorizes we came into being. From a scientific and cosmological perspective, the universe originated with the so-called Big Bang, a giant explosion of energy that created all matter. Before the Big Bang the universe existed as boundless and undifferentiated energy. Within this limitless energy were the seeds for infinite possibilities of creation. That energy still exists and is known in Jin Shin Jyutsu as the *ninth depth*. Each of us is still unified with the ninth depth; each of us is still connected, as it were, to that original potential of pure energy.

The process by which this universal energy individuates itself and becomes manifest is referred to as *densing down*. In densing down the life energy undergoes various stages of contraction in order to appear as matter. This process of contraction begins at the *eighth depth*. The eighth depth is often referred to as the *dot*. This conveys the image of a point where the vast, unbounded energy of the ninth depth begins to concentrate itself—the unknowable source of all sources.

At the *seventh depth* the life energy has condensed into "the light of the Creator." This depth provides each of us with the spark of life that animates the physical body. The image that best offers a glimpse of the seventh depth is Michelangelo's painting on the ceiling of the Sistine Chapel, in which the hand of Adam reaches out to the hand of God. Between the fingers of Adam and that of God is a little space, a synapse, across which the spark of life leaps to bring life to the flesh. The seventh depth is also associated with the sun and light.

From the sixth to first depths, the life energy denses down into the various aspects of the human form. As such, each of these depths encompasses all of the spiritual, physical, and psychological functions of our human experience. On the physical plane, for example, each depth is responsible for the creation and maintenance of a particular set of organ functions.

Each of these six depths also corresponds with a particular *attitude*. In Jin Shin Jyutsu the term *attitude* refers to a fixed emotional response, such as habitual fear or anger. The inflexible, unyielding nature of attitudes is a primary source of disharmony. Consequently, when a particular attitude becomes predominant, its related depth becomes unbalanced. This imbalance, of course, may negatively affect the particular organ function that is governed by that depth.

Happily for us, the converse is also true: When we balance a particular depth, we unburden ourselves of its affiliated attitude, which can, in turn, correct any disharmony that may be affecting the related organ. Since each of the first six depths can be regulated by a place on our hand, balancing a depth is as easy as jumper-cabling one of our fingers or our palm.

What follows is a closer look at each of the remaining six depths. Our discussion will focus primarily upon the organs and attitudes specific to each one. However, because the depths are also related to the elements that make up the earth and the heavens, it should be noted that they have numerous other correspondences as well. Thus each of the first sixth depths is also affiliated with a particular color, planet, element, and season. The chart for each depth illustrates the full range of associations not covered by our discussion.

While referring to these charts, bear in mind that each association can clue us in to the needs within a particular depth. An extreme aversion or attraction to a specific color, a tendency toward fatigue on a particular day of the week, a strong preference or dislike for a certain taste, all call attention to an imbalance of the associated depth. For example, a chronic craving for sweets is associated with an imbalance of the first depth.

the sixth depth

This is the highest dif-

ferentiated principle

in man and is his con-

sciousness in an undi-

vided and uncondi-

tioned state.

The sixth depth is the transition between the "impersonal" universe and our own "personal" human experience. (See Figure 2.1.) Accordingly, it is the source of our personal life energy. This source nourishes all of our organs, as well as all of the materializing forms of energy within us. It supports the functions of the diaphragm and umbilicus and provides vitality to our entire being. For this reason the sixth depth is often referred to as the "total harmonizer" as it harmonizes our body, mind, and spirit with each other and with the universe.

6th depth

TOTAL HARMONIZER

function	source of life
organ	diaphragm, umbilicus
attitude	total despondency
finger	center of palm
element	primordial fire
planet	moon
astrological sign	sagittarius, capricorn
season	all seasons
day of week	monday
color	pure luminous ruby red
greatest stress	sleeping
musical tone	D

taste	all inclusive
odor	all inclusive
safety energy locks	0–26

FIGURE 2.1

When this total harmonizer becomes unbalanced, utter despondency results. On the physical plane disharmony may occur in the diaphragm and umbilicus organ functions. When the sixth depth is in balance, we feel a sense of profound peace and oneness with the universe. Harmony is brought to the related organs.

To balance the sixth depth, jumper-cable the center of the palm. (See Figure 2.2.) Remember—however you choose to hold it is fine. One of the most time-honored methods of jumper-cabling the sixth depth is that of the hands at prayer. The ancients knew that this was no mere symbolic gesture but a practical, hands-on way of achieving harmony with the universe.

At the sixth depth the universal life energy has densed down to become the "blueprint" that determines the building of our manifested form. This progresses

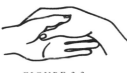

FIGURE 2.2

from our outermost surface, governed by the first depth, to our innermost physical core, governed by the fifth depth. We will now examine each of those depths in that order.

the first depth

The sustainer of the

material form.

The first depth is responsible for receiving and processing sustenance. (See Figure 2.3.) It enables us to take in nourishment from both external and internal sources. The first depth then assists us in digesting these nutrients, which are as varied as the food that we eat to the thoughts that we think.

1st depth

SUSTENANCE

function	skin surface
organ	spleen, stomach
attitude	worry
finger	thumb
element	earth
planet	saturn
astrological sign	cancer, gemini
season	hottest time of summer
day of week	saturday
color	yellow
greatest stress	sitting
musical tone	G
taste	sweet
odor	fragrant
safety energy locks	1–4

FIGURE 2.3

Appropriately, the organs associated with the first depth are the spleen and the stomach. These organs are direct expressions of this first-depth function. The stomach, of course, helps us to digest food. Additionally, the spleen is the body's source of "solar energy," which serves to energize all of the other organs. The first depth also creates our skin surface, which, through its enormous porous network, receives nutrients that come into contact with it. It is also the means by which we perceive touch and nurturing from others.

When the first depth is in harmony, we feel secure in our capacity to admit nourishment. The opposite feeling is worry, the attitude associated with an imbalance of the first depth.

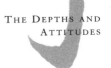

To balance the first depth, jumper-cable either thumb. (See Figure 2.4.)

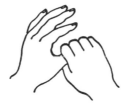

FIGURE 2.4

"WHILE RECEIVING A Jin Shin Jyutsu session from Mary, I commented on a peculiar burning sensation running down my arms and into my hands. I wanted to know what caused it. In response to my question, Mary held my hands up and invited me to take a look at my thumbs. She pointed out how arched their top joints were. 'This is the sign of a good worrier,' she told me. Mary continued to jumper-cable me. Within minutes I was again instructed to look at my thumbs. This time, to my amazement, they had straightened out! (They have remained so twelve years later.)

"THAT EVENING WHEN I returned to my hotel room, I found myself thinking about all the things that would normally provoke me to worry. But somehow, I managed to remain calm and relaxed while thinking about them.

"SINCE THAT EXPERIENCE, I have learned the value of keeping my thumbs in order. When I find myself obsessing (a less frequent occurrence), I hold my thumbs. I am still surprised by how effective they are for relaxing me."

the second depth

| Rhythm and harmony.

The second depth gives vitality and energy to the body. (See Figure 2.5.) It also moderates the essential rhythms of life—our outflow and intake. When the second depth is harmonized, we are better able to let go and receive energy at an even, unhurried rate. For this reason, the second depth is also referred to as "the little breath of life."

2nd depth

ESSENTIAL RHYTHMS OF LIFE

function	deep skin
organ	lung, large intestine
attitude	grief
finger	ring
element	air (metal)
planet	venus (uranus)
astrological sign	aries, taurus
season	fall
day of week	friday
color	white
greatest stress	reclining
musical tone	E
taste	pungent
odor	fleshy
safety energy locks	5–15

FIGURE 2.5

Not surprisingly, the second depth orchestrates the body's respiratory system. Its related organ is the lung, as well as the large intestine. Here also is where the life energy creates what is called the "deep skin" tissue, the network of tissue that underlies the skin and sheaths the body's major organs.

When we are overwhelmed by grief, the second depth is unbalanced. Grief, of course, arises out of a disruption to our natural emotional rhythms. When we grieve, we experience a diminished capacity for letting go. We become stuck, clinging to something we can't possess. Balancing the second depth helps us to release our grip on the old and be receptive to the new, on both the emotional and the physical plane (lungs and large intestine function).

To balance the second depth, jumper-cable the ring finger. (See Figure 2.6.)

"MY FRIEND HAD a twenty-year history of asthma. I showed her how to hold her ring fingers to strengthen her respiratory functions. She remarked on being able to breathe more freely after holding them and decided to receive some Jin Shin Jyutsu sessions from me. I focused on balancing the second depth. After three sessions, she said she felt like a new person. She didn't need any medication or vaporizers since receiving Jin Shin Jyutsu. Also, she said she could feel her lungs become more clear for the first time."

FIGURE 2.6

the third depth

The key to harmoniz-

ing the elements.

Like the sixth depth, the third depth is also a harmonizer. But where the sixth depth regulates our harmony with the universe, the third depth modulates the body's own inner harmony. (See Figure 2.7.) The third depth is responsible for maintaining all of the body's individual elements in the correct proportions. Similarly, the third depth harmonizes all of our various emotions. When this occurs, we are able to view life with a more compassionate eye.

3rd depth
HARMONIZER FOR ALL THE ELEMENTS

function	blood essence
organ	liver, gall bladder
attitude	anger
finger	middle
element	"key" (wood)
planet	jupiter
astrological sign	pisces, aquarius
season	spring
day of week	thursday
color	green
greatest stress	reading
musical tone	C
taste	sour
odor	rancid
safety energy locks	16–22

FIGURE 2.7

The third depth oversees the liver and gall bladder functions. It is also where the "blood essence" is created by the life energy. Fittingly, Jin Shin Jyutsu sees the blood as a harmonizing force, due to its role in distributing various nutrients to the many different parts of the body.

The attitude associated with the third depth is *anger.* Jin Shin Jyutsu sees anger as a force that can separate the soul from the body because it creates such an intense, destabilizing energy within.

When we balance the third depth, we increase our capacity for compassion as well as reinstate harmony to the liver and gall bladder functions.

To balance the third depth, simply jumper-cable one of the middle fingers. (See Figure 2.8.)

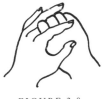

FIGURE 2.8

"My HUSBAND RETURNED *home from work in an extremely frustrated state. Everything that could have gone wrong that day did. He proceeded to tell me about the many annoyances he was subjected to.*

"As HE WAS *no stranger to Jin Shin Jyutsu, I simply suggested that he take hold of his middle finger while he spoke with me. This he did. Within a few minutes his demeanor shifted. He started to laugh as he told me, 'I can't talk about these things now—they just don't seem to bother me anymore!'"*

the fourth
depth

| The liquid of life.

The fourth depth represents "flow," or fluidity of motion. (See Figure 2.9.) It enables us to overcome the negative impact of mental, emotional, or physical stagnation.

4th depth

FLOW

function	muscular system
organ	kidney, bladder
attitude	fear
finger	index
element	water
planet	mercury (neptune, pluto)
astrological sign	scorpio, libra
season	winter
day of week	wednesday
color	blue, black
greatest stress	standing
musical tone	F
taste	salty
odor	putrid
safety energy locks	23

FIGURE 2.9

Because fluidity and motion are so central to the fourth depth, it is fitting that this depth is responsible for the creation of the muscular system. The fourth depth also governs those organs that regulate the movement of water throughout the body, namely, the kidney and bladder. Jin Shin Jyutsu, like several other ancient healing arts, believes that the kidneys also serve the larger function of storing and distributing the life energy for the entire body.

When the fourth depth becomes unbalanced, the resultant attitude is fear. Jin Shin Jyutsu defines fear as False Evidence Appearing Real. It is the source of all other attitudes. Moreover, fear is a paralyzing force that hinders the natural-motion principles of the fourth depth. It has the effect of slowing down the circulation of bodily fluids. This is not surprising when we recall that our fluid circulation is governed by the fourth-depth organs, the kidney and bladder. Balancing the fourth depth restores freedom of circulation and gives us freedom from fear.

To balance the fourth depth, jumper-cable either index finger. (See Figure 2.10.)

"I HAD A great deal of fear about an upcoming business trip. My left low back began causing me increasing pain, to such an extent, I wondered whether it would be possible to go on my trip. I went to a chiropractor to be adjusted, but my back still hurt. Finally, I boarded the plane for my trip, with my back still causing me a great deal of pain. As I sat in the plane, Mary's words came through loud and clear—'Keep it simple—when your back hurts, simply hold on to your index finger.' I held my index finger, feeling my fears melt away, and to my surprise, so did my back pain. Throughout the entire week of my trip, my back was pain free—and I was reminded of the simplicity of the Art of Jin Shin Jyutsu."

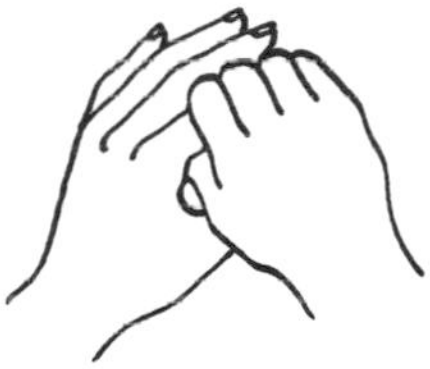

FIGURE 2.10

the fifth depth

Being in the state of

knowing instead of

just thinking.

The fifth depth is the source of our intuitive knowledge. (See Figure 2.11.) When the fifth depth is balanced, we are able to receive inspiration directly from the universe. Here, the densing-down life energy is responsible for the creation of our skeletal system. The organ functions supported by the fifth depth are the heart and small intestine. The heart, in fact, offers us an excellent insight into the essence of the fifth depth, for when our heart is open, we trust in, and are thus receptive to, the inspiration of the universe.

5th depth
INTUITIVE KNOWLEDGE

function	skeletal
organ	heart, small intestine
attitude	trying-to, pretense
finger	little
element	fire
planet	mars
astrological sign	leo, virgo
season	summer
day of week	tuesday
color	red
greatest stress	walking
musical tone	A
taste	bitter
odor	burnt
safety energy locks	24–26

FIGURE 2.11

The attitude associated with the fifth depth is pretense. Jin Shin Jyutsu refers to pretense as "trying-to." In order to prevent the fifth depth from becoming unbalanced, Jin Shin Jyutsu advises us to avoid the following common, everyday traps:

• No judging or being judged. When we make judgments, we assume that we know a situation in its totality, which is impossible on the face of it. Also, judgments assume that any situation a person finds himself in could have been avoided by that person. This is unrealistic. Each act that one undertakes represents an awareness at a particular stage of development.

- No comparing or competing. All comparisons are false. Every person and situation is unique and therefore cannot be compared with anyone or anything else. All comparisons and all forms of competition are essentially founded on illusion.

- No labeling or being labeled. To label is to limit. To be labeled by another person compromises our life condition. When we label a situation or condition with our own diagnosis, we give credibility and attention to the disharmony rather than the harmony.

- No asking why. All maturity and development is an organic process, an orderly unfolding. When we reach the time when understanding is needed, the answer emerges.

Fifth-depth imbalances often appear in the body in the form of heart or small intestine function disharmonies. Balancing the fifth depth enables us to address these physical disharmonies as well as progress beyond the "trying-to" attitude.

To balance the fifth depth, jumper-cable the little finger. (See Figure 2.12.) You may hold either one, in whatever way is most comfortable for you.

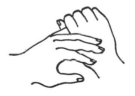

FIGURE 2.12

"IN THE EARLY 1980s, a general practitioner was sufficiently concerned about what he heard through the stethoscope to refer me to a cardiologist. My childhood diagnosis of

heart murmur was subsequently rediagnosed as aortic valve insufficiency.

"ANNUALLY, EVER SINCE, *I have received an echocardiogram, consistently demonstrating an ongoing enlargement of critical heart measurements. The cardiologist originally informed me that there was a statistical possibility of my undergoing valve replacement surgery at some point in my life. Based upon the echo indications and a cardiac catheterization in the fall of 1994, the prognosis became 'when,' not 'if' the replacement surgery would occur.*

"ENTER JIN SHIN *Jyutsu in December 1994. Since that time, I have had Jin Shin Jyutsu sessions at one- or two-week intervals. I have also dutifully practiced 'self-help' daily, giving a full five minutes each self-help session to the one 'hold' that is particularly geared toward heart function (my little finger).*

"WHEN I HAD *the fall 1995 echocardiogram, the results indicated a* diminution *in measurements that equaled the results of a full three years prior in some key measurements. This was the first incidence of reduced measurements since I began the annual echocardiogram about thirteen years ago.*

"THE CARDIOLOGIST STATED *that he had no explanation for these results. I do.*"

As we have just seen, the simple act of holding a finger can be a powerful tool for harmonizing the organ functions and neutralizing the negative influence of attitudes. When we use it in conjunction with the breath exercise at the end of Chapter 1, we greatly energize our ability to unload even the most stubbornly entrenched attitudes. Remember, nothing is more basic than breathing for the purpose of releasing attitudes and restoring harmony to mind, body, and spirit.

The breath is also essential for directing the life energy to flow in a specific pattern. With every exhalation, energy moves down the front of the body. With every subsequent inhalation, it moves up the back. As we shall see in the next chapter, this particular pattern of movement is the most elemental of all the body's energy flows. When we relax, exhale, and receive the breath, we keep this most important energy pathway free from obstruction.

the trinity flows

chapter three

*T*he simple breath and jumper-cable

exercises presented in the first two

chapters are powerful lifelong tools for

both attaining and maintaining harmony.

All of the spiritual, psychological, and

physical functions of our existence can be

regulated through our breath and fingers.

In fact, Jiro Murai's research revealed

that each one of our fingers affects 14,400

functions within the body!

43

In a sense, there is nothing else we need to know to deal with any conceivable disharmony that might occur within us. Although Jin Shin Jyutsu encompasses many other concepts and practices that we have yet to learn, they do not necessarily enable us to "do more." Yet expanding our awareness of Jin Shin Jyutsu brings a corresponding increase in our awareness of ourselves. We grow more finely attuned to the sources of disharmony. Additionally, some of the more specific exercises of Jin Shin Jyutsu can be especially beneficial for our particular personal needs. Since many of these sequences work directly upon the body's flows, we shall now pause and explore this very important concept.

what is
a flow?

During the course of his research, Jiro Murai verified that the body is traversed by energy pathways, or flow patterns. These *flows* integrate and unify all the seemingly disparate parts of the body.

In order to better understand this concept, visualize the energy as water. Water in the atmosphere is generally diffuse, taking the form of vapor. When water vapor condenses, it becomes rain and falls to earth. This, as we have already seen, is not unlike the way energy denses down through the depths.

When rainwater reaches the earth, it runs down hills and mountains into valleys, where it is channeled into rivers. The largest and mightiest of these rivers could be termed ancestral, having traveled the same course for many thousands of years. Eventually, these ancestral rivers branch off.

All of these rivers do more than simply flow endlessly, without purpose. When they run easily and abundantly, they deliver life-giving water and nutrients to the river bottom and the surrounding banks. The nearby areas become fertile. On the other hand, when their flow is too constricted or too turbulent, they do not nurture their surroundings in the same way.

Our body's energy flows operate in a similar fashion. When energy circulates easily and abundantly, body, mind, and spirit are all nourished. But when the flow becomes blocked, constricted, or stagnant, disharmony results.

In Jin Shin Jyutsu, there are three main harmonizing flows, which are collectively referred to as *the Trinity*. These three flows are the Main Central Flow and the (left and right) Supervisor Flows. The Trinity Flows are like the body's ancestral rivers. The most important of them is the Main Central Flow.

main central:
the source of life

| The oval, all inclusive, the
| rootless root of all.

In the preceding section, we compared the Main Central Flow to a mighty ancestral river. The Main Central is also like a sensitive and powerful antenna that connects us directly to the universal source of energy. This connection, as we recall, occurs within the sixth depth, where the universal life energy begins to form the source of our personal life energy. From this source the life energy flows in an oval circuit, descending the face, neck, and sternum, through the abdominal area and pubic bone, ascending the spine, and going forward over the head, then back down again.

Just as the sixth depth is the total harmonizer, the Main Central is the primary harmonizing energy flow in the body. It maintains our connection to the Creator. Accordingly, it keeps us in rhythm and harmony with the source of life.

Because of its direct connection to the original source, the Main Central Flow is the main energy source of the body. It recharges us and revitalizes all of the body's other flows. Whenever energy is unbalanced on one side or the other, the Main Central can harmonize it and bring it all back into balance.

We saw, at the end of Chapter 2, how regulating our breath directs the flow of the Main Central. Let's take a moment now to focus again on the breath. As you exhale, imagine the energy moving down the center of the front of your body. Now inhale, and visualize it moving up through the center of your back. Continue to picture this for a few moments. Envision the energy moving in a constant, unbroken circle as you breathe. This, of course, is precisely how the energy does move when you breathe. What you have just visualized is the path of the Main Central.

The Main Central pathway reveals two important concepts of Jin Shin Jyutsu. These are, respectively, the descending and ascending energy functions.

The descending energy moves down the front of the body. It helps release stagnations that occur above the waistline. Keeping the descending energy flowing is therefore useful for preventing headaches or breathing difficulties.

Conversely, the ascending energy, which moves up the back of the body, is responsible for clearing tension below the waistline. Swollen ankles, stiff hips, and bunions are but a few examples of ascending energy needs.

PROJECT 1: HARMONIZING WITH THE SOURCE OF LIFE

Sometimes certain places along the Main Central Flow become blocked or stuck. When this occurs, you can easily remove these blockages by jumper-cabling various key areas along its pathway. The following simple sequence shows how to remove those blockages and keep this most important energy "river" flowing freely.

These sequences are called *projects* because projects are creative solutions to life's problems. Problems are limited; projects are open-ended and can be fun. Here is a project that will harmonize the most important flow in the body, the Main Central, and put you back in rhythm with the universal harmony.

Remember: As you use this sequence for yourself or another person, don't be concerned with technique. Just hold each area for a couple of minutes, or until you feel a rhythmic pulse. (See Figure 3.1.)

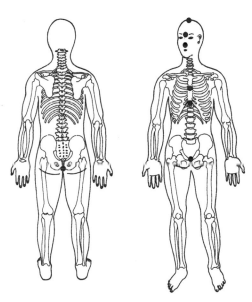

FIGURE 3.1

1. Begin by placing your right palm or fingers or fingertips on the top of the head. Hold your right hand there throughout the remainder of the exercise (until Step 7, when you will move it to the base of the spine).

2. Place your left finger or fingers between the eyebrows. This will revitalize the deep body energy circulation (energy deep inside the body), improve memory, and dissipate mental stress and even senility.

3. Place your left hand on the tip of the nose. This will revitalize the reproductive functions and the superficial body energy circulation.

4. Place your left fingertips on the sternum or breastbone. This will revitalize the lungs, breathing, pelvic girdle, and

hips. (Just a reminder: Your right hand remains on the top of the head.)

5. Place your left fingertips at the base of the sternum, directly above the solar plexus. This will revitalize the Source of Life energy, both descending and ascending.

6. Place your left fingertips over the top of the pubic bone. This will revitalize the descending Source of Life energy and strengthen the spine.

7. Leave your left hand on top of the pubic bone. Remove the fingertips of your right hand from the top of the head and place them at the base of the spine, at the area of the coccyx. (The palm or back of the right hand may be used, whichever is more comfortable for you.) The last placement of the hands revitalizes the ascending Source of Life energy and aids in circulation of the legs and feet.

"MY HUSBAND, A medical doctor, had recurring back problems for many years, which he had treated chiropractically and through various kinds of massage. Finally, last summer his lower back totally rebelled and gave out. He slipped the disc of his fourth lumbar vertebra. For weeks he lived in great pain and fear: fear of excruciating pain, fear of having to have an operation. I worked on him sporadically for a few weeks when I had time, and he experienced some relief. But he was still worried and frightened, in a great deal of pain, and unable to move freely. Desperately, we sent the kids away for one long weekend, and I was determined to treat him twice a day for the duration. While treating him so intensely, I found myself utilizing the Main Central Flow because it runs through the center of the body, energizing the spine and total being. Through using this flow, we were able to

strengthen and straighten the spine and relieve pressure on the disc. That weekend was the turning point for him. Afterward he felt he could see the light at the end of the tunnel, that he was actually on the road to full recovery."

the supervisor flows

The illuminating intelligence of

the body.

Along with the Main Central Flow, the left and right Supervisor Flows constitute the Trinity. Both Supervisor Flows are born out of the Main Central. At the base of the spine, the Main Central branches off into two flows that run down the inside of each leg. At the inside of each knee, these branches become the Supervisor Flows. As the name implies, each of these flows then serves to "supervise" all of the functions on their respective sides of the body.

The left and right Supervisor Flows are mirror images of each other, existing like two vertical ovals of energy on each side of the body. The left Supervisor Flow flows down and up the center of the left side of the body. The right Supervisor Flow follows a similar pathway along the center of the right side of the body.

Each time the Supervisor Flow begins its circuit anew at the knee, the energy travels a little deeper. In this way the energy conveyed by the Supervisor Flow is distributed throughout all five depths of the body.

The following project enables you to balance either the left or the right Supervisor Flow. It is especially useful for clearing the head and breathing, aiding digestion, and easing back stress.

PROJECT 2: THE SUPERVISOR FLOWS

Because the left and right Supervisor
Flows oversee all of the bodily functions
along their respective sides, you can apply
the appropriate Supervisor Flow when one
side or the other feels particularly tense.

For *left-side* descending energy needs (see
Figure 3.2):

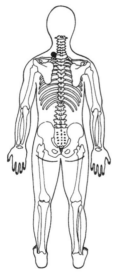

FIGURE 3.2

1. Place your right hand on the left
   shoulder.

2. Hold the left buttock with your left
   hand.

For *left-side* ascending energy needs (see
Figure 3.3):

FIGURE 3.3

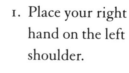

1. Place your right
   hand on the left
   shoulder.

2. Hold the left
   groin with your
   left hand.

For *right-side* de-
scending energy needs
(see Figure 3.4):

1. Place your left hand on the right shoulder.

2. Hold the right buttock with your right hand.

For *right-side* ascending energy needs
(see Figure 3.5):

1. Place your left hand on the right
   shoulder.

2. Hold the right groin with your right
   hand.

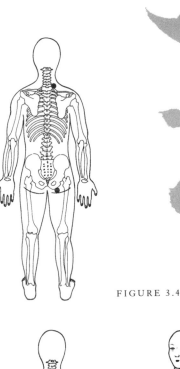

FIGURE 3.4

*"SHARYN AND I have known each
other since we were three years old,
and we were born exactly two
months apart. As we grew and played
together, my mother noticed a
dissimilarity in our development. It
was found that Sharyn had scoliosis.
After five years of wearing a chin-to-
sacrum brace, an operation was
performed at age fourteen, and a metal
rod was attached to the length of
Sharyn's spine. In 1993, I went to visit
Sharyn in Seattle. We had a lot of
catching up to do, as it had been eight
years since we had seen each other. I was
shocked to see her limping; I never
remembered her limping. When we
arrived at her home, I asked her to
stand, and I felt for her spine. I found it
one inch left of where a spine should be.
I brought this to her attention and told her I knew of
something that might help correct the position of her spine:
Jin Shin Jyutsu. I used a right Supervisor Flow and then a
left Supervisor Flow. Sharyn stood again, but this time
more erect—her spine seemed straighter. She no longer*

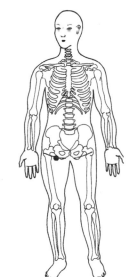

FIGURE 3.5

limped. Sharyn also noticed that her body felt more relaxed and that she could sit for longer periods of time without having to get up and move every half hour because of stiffness."

the diagonal mediator flows

The activity principle of the body.

Although the left and right Diagonal Mediator Flows are not included within the Trinity, they have an important relationship to the Trinity that cannot be overlooked. The left and right Diagonal Mediator Flows start at their respective shoulders and traverse both sides of the body from back to front, side to side, and top to bottom, ending up at the opposite-side knees. They harmonize the left and right Supervisor Flows with each other and with the Main Central Flow.

The Mediator ensures that all the flows within the body will cross at the Main Central so they may constantly receive revitalizing life energy from the Source. Also, when one side of the body becomes so tense that the other side is affected, one of the Mediator Flows can be used to bring both sides into balance. Because of these functions, it is vitally important to keep the Mediator Flows in harmony.

PROJECT 3: HARMONIZING THE MEDIATOR FLOWS

Here is a dynamic sequence that will harmonize the Mediator Flows and reduce fatigue, tension, and stress. If one side of the body seems particularly tense, utilize whichever of the following two sequences is appropriate. They can be applied at any time of day.

For left-side energy needs (see Figure 3.6):

1. Place your left thumb over the left ring fingernail. Make a circle with the pad of the thumb over the ring fingernail. (This helps to clear the chest.)

2. Place your right hand over the left shoulder. (This revitalizes the ascending energy.)

FIGURE 3.6

3. Bring the knees together so that their inner sides touch. The feet may be apart or together, whichever is more comfortable. (This revitalizes the descending energy.)

For right-side energy needs (see Figure 3.7):

1. Place your right thumb over the right ring fingernail. Make a circle with the pad of the thumb (palm side) over the ring fingernail. (This helps to clear the chest.)

2. Place your left hand over the right shoulder. (This revitalizes ascending energy.)

3. Bring the knees together so that the insides touch. The feet may be apart or together, whichever is more comfortable. (This revitalizes the descending energy.)

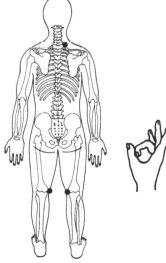

FIGURE 3.7

Note: This project can also be used for harmonizing the Supervisor Flows as well.

"I WAS COMING down with the symptoms of the flu—body aches, fever, and chills. I decided to use a Mediator self-help 'quickie' to see if I could nip it in the bud. I knew that the Mediator was effective in clearing shoulder tension, one of the underlying causes for flu and colds.

"MY LEFT SHOULDER was very tight, so I continued to hold it for nearly an hour. When it finally cleared, my fever subsided. I was able to sleep peacefully through the night. The next morning when I awoke, there were no traces of the flu, and it didn't return."

In order to emphasize the importance of the Trinity Flows, let's imagine them as rivers again. The Main Central would be the largest and most important, as it is the one that is fed by the original source. The left and right Supervisor Flows are its two major branches, diverting water/energy from the main river to the outlying regions. Thus, when we keep the Main Central flowing easily, its two main branches are able to receive sufficient energy to flow freely as well.

And when these two major branches flow abundantly, they, in turn, fertilize and nourish a host of other important functions. The Supervisor Flows are home to the twenty-six Safety Energy Locks. These safety energy locks, which will be examined in detail in the following chapters, can function like little dams. When one of our energy rivers becomes obstructed, pools of excess energy begin to form. Utilizing these twenty-six safety energy locks allows us to clear these obstructions and release the pooled-up energy back into the general flow of energy throughout our being.

safety energy locks: 1–15

chapter four

Numbers are qualities, not quantities.

As we have seen, our health and harmony are dependent upon the constant, unobstructed passage of the life energy throughout our being. Thus far we have focused upon the stages by which this energy manifests itself within us (the depths) and upon the major pathways by which it travels through us (the Trinity Flows). These concepts form the foundation of Jin Shin Jyutsu. Our

55

increased awareness of them is essential for the maintenance of our overall balance and well-being.

Sometimes excess energy becomes stuck at a particular area within us. We can easily release this energy using the twenty-six sites known as safety energy locks. The safety energy locks are also called the "keys to the kingdom" because they "unlock" the flow of life energy within the body, mind, and spirit. When the safety energy locks are open, energy flows smoothly throughout our being. However, as we abuse ourselves mentally, emotionally, or physically through the course of our daily routines, our "braking" or safety energy lock system becomes activated. Thus, the safety energy locks serve as a kind of early warning system that lets us know when certain parts of our system have become overloaded. If we heed the friendly warning, we can instantly help ourselves and prevent further discomfort or misery. By familiarizing ourselves with the safety energy locks, we can root out the causes of imbalances. Restoring harmony can be simply a matter of applying our hands to unlock particular safety energy locks.

The twenty-six safety energy locks (SELs) are arranged in pairs on each side of the body, so that there are twenty-six on the left side and twenty-six on the right. Each set is a mirror image of the other. (See Figure 4.1.) This arrangement, of course, roughly corresponds with the location of the left and right Supervisor Flows, discussed in the previous chapter. Not surprisingly, all twenty-six of the safety energy locks are located within the Supervisor Flows.

When we explored the Supervisor Flows, we noted that one of their functions is to carry its energy to all five of the body's depths. Since all of the SELs are located along the Supervisor Flows, we can understand that each depth would also house its own particular set of SELs.

When you heighten your awareness of the relationships between the depths and the safety energy locks, you will take yet another step toward regaining your sense of wholeness, of the interelatedness of all the various parts of yourself. Familiarizing yourself with these different relationships will give you an increased versatility in your approach to any number of disharmonies that might arise within.

As we have seen, each of the first five depths is responsible for a specific set of functions encompassing body, mind, and spirit. We have seen how to balance each of these depths using the hands. Now we will see that opening a particular safety energy lock also helps us to keep its related depth in balance, since each of the twenty-six safety energy locks facilitates a particular depth. Conversely, when we harmonize a specific depth, we strengthen the safety energy locks associated with that depth. The associations between the depths and the SELs can be summarized as follows:

- The first depth is associated with Safety Energy Locks 1 through 4.

- The second depth is associated with Safety Energy Locks 5 through 15.

- The third depth is associated with Safety Energy Locks 16 through 22.

- The fourth depth is associated with Safety Energy Lock 23.

- The fifth depth is associated with Safety Energy Locks 24 through 26.

- The sixth depth is considered all-inclusive, meaning that it serves as a harmonizer for the total being.

In the ensuing discussion we will examine the twenty-six safety energy locks within the context of their associated depths. In this chapter we will look at Safety Energy Locks 1 through 15, which are contained within the first and second depths.

In this overview, we will focus on the location and universal meaning of each safety energy lock (SEL). In addition, we will learn the specific disharmonies that can arise when a particular SEL becomes "locked," as well as some easy-to-use exercises. For jumper-cabling the safety energy locks, we use the same guidelines that we have been using throughout—hold comfortably for a few minutes or until a pulsation can be felt. There is no need to be overly concerned with precision. There is a three-inch effective radius around every safety energy lock. In time, as one's awareness grows, one may learn to "bull's-eye," but this is not essential. For convenience, the accompanying index can help you locate specific safety energy locks that may be used for addressing particular needs.

Index of Safety Energy Locks

TO HELP:	USE SEL:	TO HELP:	USE SEL:
Abdomen	1, 15, 23	Fever	3
Ankle	9, 15, 17	Foot	9, 15
Appetite	13	Head	1, 7, 16, 18
Arm	9, 11, 12	Heart	10, 15, 17
Back	2, 6, 9, 19	Hip	6, 9, 11, 14
Bloat	1, 15, 17	Insomnia	4, 18
Brain	23	Knee	10, 15
Breast	17, 19	Leg	2, 9, 11, 15
Breathing	1, 2, 3	Mental Clarity	7, 20, 21, 25
Chest	6, 9, 10, 13	Muscles	8, 16
Circulation	10, 23	Neck	11, 12, 13, 16
Colds	3	Nervous System	17
Convulsions	7	Pelvis	3, 8
Digestion	2, 5, 7, 19	Reproductive	8, 13, 16, 17
Dizziness	21	Shakiness	24, 26
Ear	5, 20	Shoulder	10, 11, 13
Elimination	8, 16	Throat	3, 4, 10
Emotional Equilibrium	12, 22, 23, 24	Thyroid	14
Equilibrium	6, 20	Weight	21
Eye	4, 20	Wrist	9, 11

While reading the following summaries of the safety energy locks, please refer to Figure 4.1 to find their location. Some of the safety energy locks are located on the back or in other places that are hard to reach if you are jumper-cabling yourself. For self-help purposes, Jiro Murai discovered that there are corresponding areas throughout the body that are within easy reach. Thus, any one of us can open all of our own safety energy locks with relative ease.

Along similar lines, you will note that many of the following exercises involve jumper-cabling two different SELs at the same time. The additional SEL serves as a sort of "outlet," which helps channel the energy freed up from the "locked" SEL.

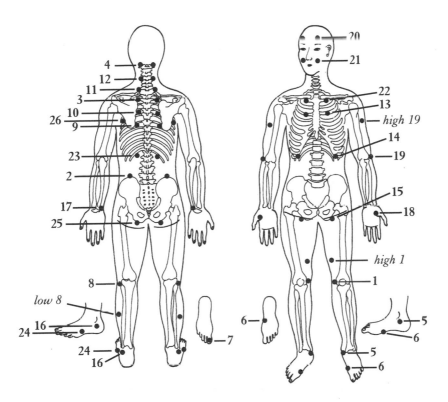

FIGURE 4.1

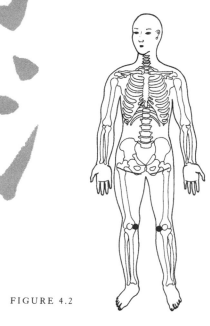

FIGURE 4.2

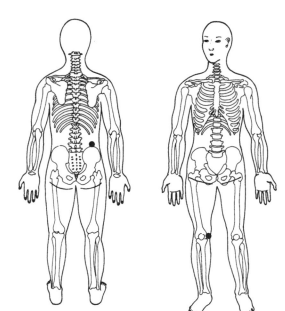

FIGURE 4.3

the first-depth
SELs (1–4)

SAFETY ENERGY LOCK 1: THE PRIME MOVER

Safety Energy Lock 1 is located on the inside of each knee, right at the bulge, where the thigh and shinbone connect. (See Figure 4.2.) SEL 1 unifies the descending energy (which travels down the front of the body) with the ascending energy (which flows up the back) and thus harmonizes us from head to toe. SEL 1 is considered *"the prime mover, connecting extreme heights with extreme depths."*

Opening Safety Energy Lock 1 helps all forms of abdominal distress (bloating, discomfort) and headaches. It also promotes deeper and easier breathing.

You can jumper-cable either yourself or another person by applying your hands—the thumb, fingers, palm, or back of your hand. After holding the left and right knees at the medial or inner side for a few minutes, you will gradually feel the discomfort fade away.

You can also help SEL 1 by jumper-cabling it in conjunction with Safety Energy Lock 2:

1. Place your left hand on the right knee, at Safety Energy Lock 1, and

your right hand on the right hip, at Safety Energy Lock 2.
(See Figure 4.3.)

2. Place your right hand on the left knee, at Safety Energy
   Lock 1, and your left hand on the left hip, at Safety Energy
   Lock 2.

"*I WAS STAYING in a beautiful home off Kahlua Bay. I was
excited to go to the ocean for my daily swim. There had been
a huge storm the night before, and when I got to the beach,
the water looked different. It was murky, not the crystal-clear
turquoise that it usually was. Being an avid swimmer, I went
right on in alone.*

"*I SWAM OUT about fifty yards, and I felt this sharp electrical
current running through my body. I started to go numb, and I
panicked. I somehow made my way to the shore. I had been
wrapped by a man-of-war jellyfish. Its long tentacles wrapped
around my face, neck, chest, waist, and thighs. I began
rubbing my skin with sand to remove the gelatinous stinging
substance, and then my heart started to race and I could not
catch my breath, and my body began to shake uncontrollably.
I thought for a minute, 'Oh, my God, I'm going to die!' I lay
in the sand and grabbed my ones (the inside of each knee)
with my hands crossed, and I held on for dear life.*

"*MARY'S DESCRIPTION OF the number one was the only thing
I could remember, the prime mover, and I felt like I needed to
move this out of my body fast. I held on until about twenty
minutes later. Finally, I felt it subside in my body, and I was
able to walk home. My friends greeted me at the door. I was
covered in welts, and they were ready to take me to the
hospital. I lay in bed instead and did my Jin Shin Jyutsu self-
help, and I was much better by the next day.*"

SAFETY ENERGY LOCK 2: WISDOM

Safety Energy Lock 2 is located in the lower back, at the top of the hip-bone, on the left and right sides of the body. (See Figure 4.4.) SEL 2 is associated with the life force for all creatures and with wisdom. When SEL 2 is opened, we reconnect with the original wisdom and purpose for living.

Safety Energy Lock 2 can be used to relieve all forms of back discomfort. It balances digestion and breathing. It also reduces tension and stress in the legs.

To jumper-cable, apply the hands directly on the left and right SEL 2s, right on the top of the pelvic bone on the back. Or jumper-cable Safety Energy Locks 2 and 3 together, as follows:

1. Place your left hand on the right shoulder, at Safety Energy Lock 3, and your right hand on the right hip, at Safety Energy Lock 2. (See Figure 4.5.)

2. Place your right hand on the left shoulder, at Safety Energy Lock 3, and your left hand on the left hip, at Safety Energy Lock 2.

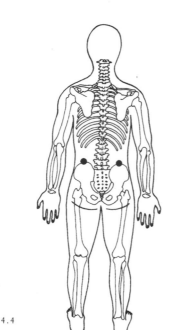

FIGURE 4.4

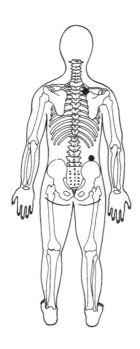

FIGURE 4.5

SAFETY ENERGY LOCK 3: THE DOOR

Safety Energy Lock 3 is located on the upper back, by the inside and upper corners of the shoulder blades, to the left and right of the spine. (See Figure 4.6.) SEL 3 functions like a door, swinging forth to unload tension, then swinging back to receive purified energy.

Safety Energy Lock 3 is jumper-cabled to aid in breathing, to treat fevers, colds, and sore throats, and to boost the body's immune system by releasing its own natural antibiotic. It is also a good safety energy lock to jumper-cable when there is stress and tension in the pelvic girdle. Apply your right hand to the left SEL 3 and the left hand to the right SEL 3, and feel the tension quickly dissipate.

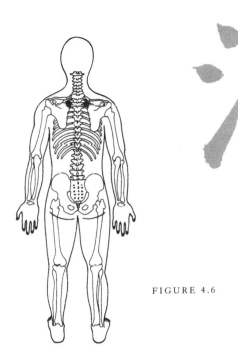

FIGURE 4.6

You can also jumper-cable SEL 3 together with SEL 15, using this simple sequence:

1. Place your left hand on the right shoulder, at Safety Energy Lock 3, and your right hand on the right groin, at Safety Energy Lock 15. (See Figure 4.7.)

2. Place your right hand on the left shoulder, at Safety Energy Lock 3, and your left hand on the left groin, at Safety Energy Lock 15.

"ON A FLIGHT from Salt Lake City to South Dakota, a young mother was seated near me with a six-month-old infant. The mother was visibly distressed because her baby was running a

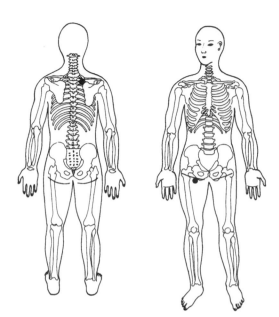

FIGURE 4.7

very high fever of 105 degrees. Two doses of aspirin had failed to reduce the child's fever.

"THE MOTHER EVENTUALLY became so upset that the pilots decided to schedule an emergency landing in Wyoming. In the interim, one of the stewardesses asked if there was anyone on board who could help in some way. I went over to the child and jumper-cabled her threes, remembering that it is a natural antibiotic and good for reducing fevers. After about twenty minutes or so, the plane landed in Wyoming. Upon landing, the mother took her baby's temperature and was relieved to see that it had already dropped three degrees, to 102!"

SAFETY ENERGY LOCK 4: THE WINDOW

Safety Energy Lock 4 is located at the base of the skull, at the occipital ridge (on the left and right). (See Figure 4.8.) It is called the "window" that lets in the light of knowledge and life-giving breath.

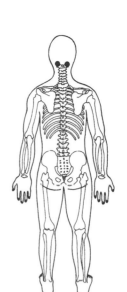

Safety Energy Lock 4 harmonizes eye and throat discomforts. Jumper-cable the SEL 4s whenever you or a friend suffer from insomnia, from weakness or straining of the eyes, or from a sore or dry throat.

To jumper-cable SEL 4, simply hold each one with your hands for a few minutes. Or jumper-cable them while holding the cheekbones, the SELs 21:

1. Place your left hand on the right base of skull, at Safety Energy Lock 4, and your right hand on the left cheekbone, at Safety Energy Lock 21. (See Figure 4.9.)

2. Place your right hand on the left base of skull, at Safety Energy Lock 4, and your left hand on the right cheekbone, at Safety Energy Lock 21.

FIGURE 4.8

"WHILE JUMPER-CABLING a young woman, I noticed her pupils were extremely dilated. She said she had a hereditary eye disease—a progressive problem that left her with peripheral vision and very little central vision,

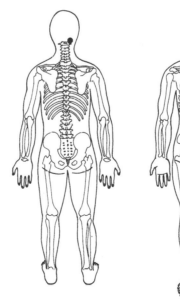

FIGURE 4.9

'but,' she said, 'nothing can help it.' I didn't say anything, but started holding her fours and got her holding them, too. A couple of weeks later, I saw her. 'Do I have something to tell you!' she said. 'I've been afraid to say anything, I'm afraid it will go away, but I've started to see. Every day I see more.' She proceeded to tell me how she had been noticing things she had never seen—architecture, etc.—and that her boyfriend was literally dragging her through the city because she would first stand and stare at the newness of everything. It was like being with Alice in Wonderland. Thank you for the gift of Jin Shin Jyutsu!"

the second-depth
SELs (5–15)

SAFETY ENERGY LOCK 5: REGENERATION

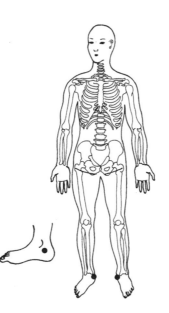

FIGURE 4.10

Located on the inside of the ankle, between the ankle bone and the heel, Safety Energy Lock 5 restores our ability to release all that is old and take up the new. (See Figure 4.10.) For this reason, it is associated with regeneration and rebirth. When SEL 5 is open, we feel liberated from all the bondage that held us back in the past. Since fear is among the greatest of all bonds, the SEL 5s are often jumper-cabled whenever we experience fear.

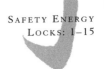

The SEL 5s are also useful for helping digestive and hearing disorders.

To jumper-cable the SEL 5s, hold the insides of each ankle, or—

if that position is too uncomfortable— place a hand on each of the SEL 15s at the groin. Opening the SEL 15s along with the SEL 3s will also open the SEL 5s:

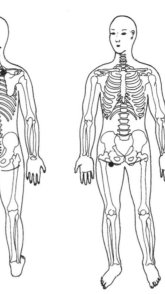

FIGURE 4.11

1. Place your right hand on the right groin, at Safety Energy Lock 15, and your left hand on the right shoulder, at Safety Energy Lock 3. (See Figure 4.11.)

2. Hold for a few minutes, then place your left hand on the left groin, at Safety Energy Lock 15, and your right hand on the left shoulder, at Safety Energy Lock 3.

SAFETY ENERGY LOCK 6:
BALANCE AND DISCRIMINATION

Safety Energy Lock 6 is associated with balance and discrimination. It is located on the arch of each foot, about midway be-

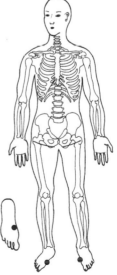

FIGURE 4.12

tween the sole side of the big toe and the end of the heel. (See Figure 4.12.) The arch is the structure that enables us to maintain a balanced position in the world. Like its physical manifestation, SEL 6 allows us to balance universal inspiration with practical groundedness.

Safety Energy Lock 6 releases tension in the chest and can be used to clear tension in the hips and back. The SEL 6s also help us gain equilibrium.

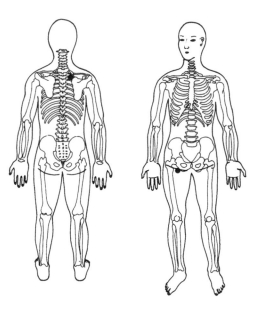

FIGURE 4.13

To jumper-cable the SEL 6s, hold the arches of each foot at the safety energy lock. Like the SEL 5s, the SEL 6s can also be opened up by jumper-cabling SEL 15 and SEL 3. The exact same sequence presented for SEL 5 is equally effective here.

1. Place your right hand on the right groin, at Safety Energy Lock 15, and your left hand on the right shoulder, at Safety Energy Lock 3. (See Figure 4.13.)

2. Hold for a few minutes, then place your left hand on the left groin, at Safety Energy Lock 15, and your right hand on the left shoulder, at Safety Energy Lock 3.

SAFETY ENERGY LOCK 7: VICTORY

Safety Energy Lock 7 is located on the underside of the big toe.

(See Figure 4.14.) Traditionally, SEL 7 is associated with development and with the completion of a spiritual cycle, hence victory.

Because it is found at the very bottom of the body, SEL 7 is associated with the very top. Therefore, it is the safety energy lock that will help clear the mind and head. The SEL 7s can relieve headaches and convulsions and are also useful for facilitating digestion.

Jumper-cable the SEL 7s by holding the big toe at the indicated place. If this is too inconvenient, the SEL 7s can also be opened by jumper-cabling the groin, at SEL 15, and the hip, at SEL 2:

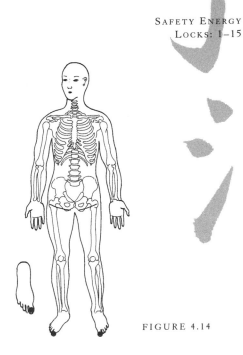

FIGURE 4.14

1. Place your left hand on the left groin, at Safety Energy Lock 15, and your right hand on the right hip, at Safety Energy Lock 2. (You can use either your palm or the back of your hand.) (See Figure 4.15.)

2. Put your right hand on the right groin, at Safety Energy Lock 15, and your left hand on the left hip, at Safety Energy Lock 2.

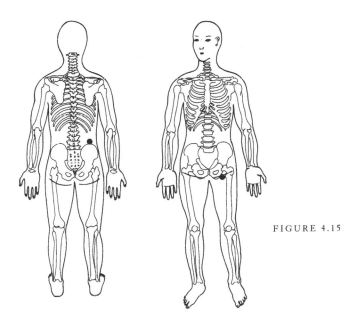

FIGURE 4.15

"I HAD EXPERIENCED grand mal seizures for eighteen years. My convulsions were extremely severe, and most of the time my seizures came upon me while I slept. I'd wake up seconds before I started convulsing. I learned from classes on Jin Shin Jyutsu that by holding my sevens, the energy blockage creating seizures could be cleared.

"ONE DAWN, AFTER an extremely stressful week, I awoke feeling the aura of a seizure upon me. Quickly, I grabbed my big toes and held them for dear life. As my body started to convulse, I tightened the grip on my toes until my knuckles turned white, so the force of the convulsions would not pull my fingers away. To my amazement, the tremor quickly abated before it reached its usual full force, and it did not render me unconscious as it always did.

"I LAY IN bed for some time, continuing to hold my big toes until I felt confident enough to sit up and get a cup of tea. After the experience, I was elated and felt that I was in control of my body for the first time in years. I was astounded that the Jin Shin Jyutsu worked so quickly and so easily."

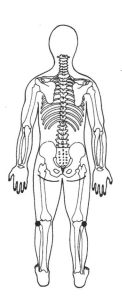

FIGURE 4.16

SAFETY ENERGY LOCK 8: RHYTHM, STRENGTH, AND PEACE

Safety Energy Lock 8 is located at the lateral side (outside) of the back of the knees. (See Figure 4.16.) When the SEL 8s are open, we experience and feel more attuned to the rhythm, strength, and peace of the universe.

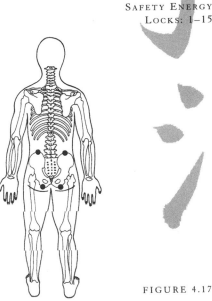

Safety Energy Lock 8 aids the elimination and reproductive functions. It is also good for the reduction of muscle tension as well as for rectum and pelvic girdle projects.

Jumper-cable the SEL 8s while sitting in a comfortable chair or lying down and bringing the knees closer to the chest. If these positions are uncomfortable, the SEL 8s may also be opened by jumper-cabling either SEL 25, at the sit-bones, or SEL 2, at the hip.

1. Place your left hand on the left buttock, at Safety Energy Lock 25, and your right hand on the right buttock, at Safety Energy Lock 25. (See Figure 4.17.)

FIGURE 4.17

2. Place your left hand on the left hip, at Safety Energy Lock 2, and your right hand on the right hip, at Safety Energy Lock 2.

SAFETY ENERGY LOCK 9:
ENDING OF ONE CYCLE, BEGINNING OF ANOTHER

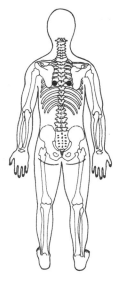

Safety Energy Lock 9 is located on the middle of the back, between the bottom of the shoulder blades and the spine. (See Figure 4.18.) Jumper-cable the SEL 9s whenever someone is having trouble clearing their slate. The SEL 9s give us inspiration to let go of the old and take up the new.

FIGURE 4.18

Safety Energy Lock 9 also connects the lower part of the body with the upper part. As such, the SEL 9s harmonize and energize the extremities. Jumper-cable them whenever there is chest congestion, an arm and back project, a sprained ankle, or hip discomfort.

Since few of us can reach the SEL 9s, we can instead hold SEL 19, which is located at the elbows, on the thumb-side crease. By opening the SEL 19s, you automatically open the SEL 9s as well.

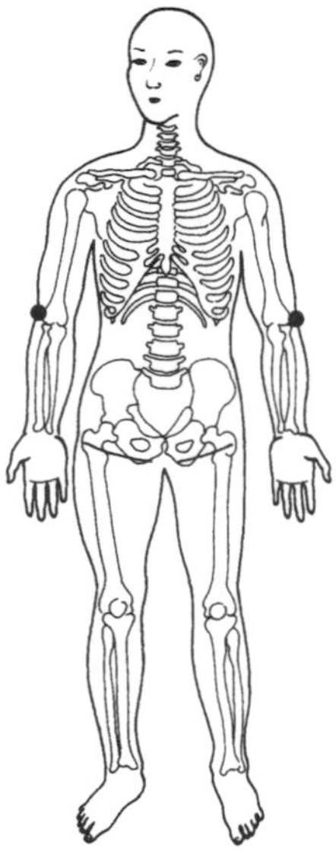

1. To clear the SEL 9s, jumper-cable SEL 19 at the elbows. Hold them at the thumb-side crease of the elbows on both arms. (See Figure 4.19.)

FIGURE 4.19

2. If it is uncomfortable to jumper-cable both elbows at the same time, you can jumper-cable the right elbow and then the left elbow in succession.

"*FOLLOWING MY FIRST class with Mary Burmeister in 1979, I eagerly recruited several friends as guinea pigs so that I might practice. One of them was a healthy male in his early forties whom I had known for twelve years. Often he had told me about his career, which was lucrative and secure but unfulfilling. He dreaded going to work but was too comfortably rooted in his job to make the changes he desired.*

"*AT THE TIME he came to me, he was seeking to rid himself of a discomfort in his arm. The nines help the arms. They also represent the end of a cycle and beginning of a new. Both seemed applicable to his situation, so I decided to concentrate on clearing his nines.*

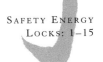

"AFTER RECEIVING SIX treatments in two weeks, he arrived at my home one morning with news. The day before, while at work, he spontaneously informed his employer that he was quitting. This decision received the full blessing of his boss, who had long thought that my friend was somehow in the wrong business."

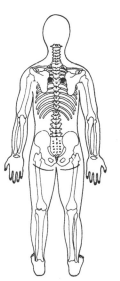

FIGURE 4.20

SAFETY ENERGY LOCK 10: WAREHOUSE OF ABUNDANCE

Safety Energy Lock 10 is located on the upper back, between the shoulder blades and the spine, in line with the middle of the shoulder blades. (See Figure 4.20.) SEL 10 is regarded as the "warehouse of abundance" because it releases an outpouring of limitless life energy when unlocked.

Releasing Safety Energy Lock 10 also harmonizes the heart, circulation, throat, voice, shoulders, and knees. Like the SEL 9s, the SEL 10s also harmonize the chest area. They are especially good for balancing the blood pressure.

Like the SEL 9s, the SEL 10s may be hard to get to. Instead of holding them directly, hold the left upper arm (known as the high SEL 19) with the right hand, and the right upper arm with the left hand, for several minutes. Or jumper-cable the upper arms with the opposite thighs (the high SEL 1s), as follows:

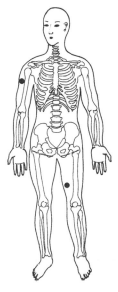

FIGURE 4.21

1. Place your left hand on the right high SEL 19 (on the upper arm), and your right hand on the left high SEL 1 (on the inner thigh). (See Figure 4.21.)

2. Place your right hand on the left high SEL 19 (on the upper arm), and your left hand on the right high SEL 1 (on the inner thigh).

SAFETY ENERGY LOCK 11: UNLOADING THE BURDENS OF THE PAST AND FUTURE

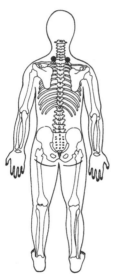

FIGURE 4.22

Safety Energy Lock 11 is located on the upper back, just below the place where the neck joins the shoulders. (See Figure 4.22.) The SEL 11s help us to unload excess baggage.

Jumper-cabling Safety Energy Lock 11 harmonizes the shoulders and neck. It is also good for easing discomfort in the hips and legs. Releasing the SEL 11s also benefits the arms, including the elbows, wrists, hands, and fingers.

The left SEL 11 is jumper-cabled by placing the right hand on it. The right SEL 11 is held with the left hand. It is also helpful to jumper-cable SEL 11 with the buttock, SEL 25, to clear SEL 11:

1. Hold the right shoulder, at Safety Energy Lock 11, with your left hand, and the right buttock, at Safety Energy Lock 25, with your right hand. (See Figure 4.23.)

2. Jumper-cable the left shoulder, at Safety Energy Lock 11, with your right hand, and hold the left buttock, at Safety Energy Lock 25, with your left hand.

"ABOUT THREE YEARS ago, I was hired to do home care for Laura, a 38-year-old woman who was bedridden, paralyzed from her chest down, and labeled with multiple sclerosis. Once a day I had to do a range of motion with her legs to prevent further deterioration. Her legs were very stiff and difficult to move. My good friend, a Jin Shin Jyutsu practitioner, showed how to hold Laura's elevens and fifteens. After holding each side for ten minutes, what a surprise! Laura's legs were limber, and I could move them very easily. I was so impressed that I decided right then to study and practice this art. The deeper I explore Jin Shin Jyutsu, the more I am impressed."

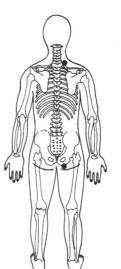

FIGURE 4.23

SAFETY ENERGY LOCK 12: NOT MY WILL BUT THY WILL

Safety Energy Lock 12 is found at the back of the neck, midway between the skull and the shoulders, on each side of the cervical vertebrae. (See Figure 4.24.) The SEL 12s have a powerful effect on our psychology because they are able to realign our will with the universal will. Opening them can restore emotional equilibrium and helps to eliminate anger. Opening the SEL 12s also helps relieve tension in the neck and arms.

Jumper-cable the SEL 12s by placing each hand on the left and right SEL ones respectively. In addition, jumper-cabling the coccyx

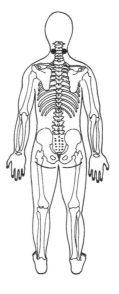

FIGURE 4.24

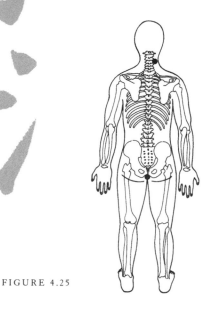

FIGURE 4.25

(at the base of spine) along with SEL 12 helps facilitate the release of stuck energy.

1. Place your left hand on the right side of the neck, at Safety Energy Lock 12, and your right hand on the base of spine, at the coccyx. (See Figure 4.25.)

2. Place your right hand on the left side of the neck, at Safety Energy Lock 12, and your left hand on the base of spine, at the coccyx.

SAFETY ENERGY LOCK 13: LOVE YOUR ENEMIES

Safety Energy Lock 13 is located on the front of the rib cage, a few inches below the clavicle, by the third rib. (See Figure 4.26.) When the SEL 13s are open, we are better able to see the good in all people, even those with whom we disagree or clash.

The SEL 13s harmonize the reproductive functions. They also help balance the appetite and can reduce tension in the shoulders and neck.

To jumper-cable the SEL 13s, simply place the hands on each one. You can also hold the high SEL 19s (on the upper arms) as follows:

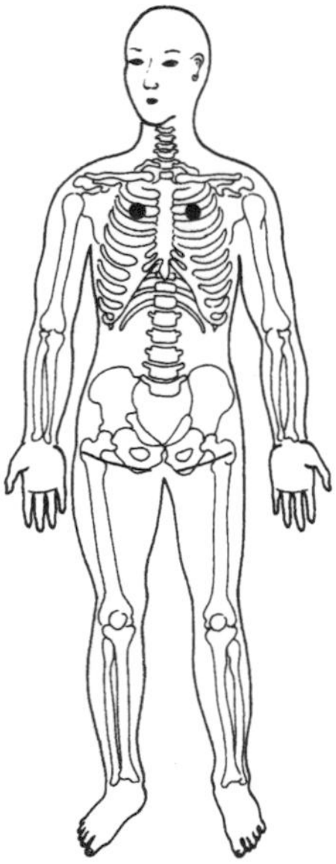

1. Place your left hand on the right upper arm. (See Figure 4.27.)

FIGURE 4.26

2. Place your right hand on the left upper arm. (You can apply this separately on each arm, or hold the left and right upper arms together.)

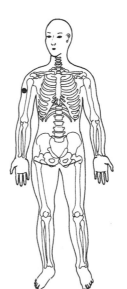

FIGURE 4.27

"A PREGNANT CO-WORKER was scheduled to have a cesarean section on Monday. Her last day at the office was the Thursday before this established due date. She told me her pregnancy had been fine, but the baby was in the wrong position for delivery. The doctor had tried several times to 'turn' the baby around, but it was still feet first.

"DEBBIE SAID SHE just wished she could go into natural labor—to know it was the baby ready to come rather than the doctors making the decision. She asked if I could apply some Jin Shin Jyutsu to her before she left that day. (This was the ONLY time I worked on her). I used a thirteen flow.

"THE NEXT DAY I received a call that Debbie had had a baby girl that morning (Friday). When I called her at the hospital she was thrilled. She had gone into labor at three A.M. on Friday morning, and the baby HAD turned around! The doctors, however, performed the cesarean anyway, as it had been the 'plan,' but Debbie recuperated very quickly, and to this day she calls her daughter her 'Jin Shin baby.' "

SAFETY ENERGY LOCK 14: EQUILIBRIUM, SUSTENANCE

Located on the front bottom of the rib cage, Safety Energy Lock 14 gives us the ability to nourish ourselves and maintain balance in everyday life. (See Figure 4.28.) We can jumper-cable the SEL 14s

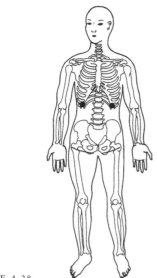

FIGURE 4.28

whenever there is disharmony or tension in either the hip or thigh region. Opening the SEL 14s also maintains equilibrium between the upper and lower body.

You can jumper-cable the SEL 14s by placing a hand on them on the left and right sides. You can also harmonize them by jumper-cabling the SEL 19s, found by the crease of the elbows (on the thumb side), as follows:

1. Place your left hand on the right elbow, at Safety Energy Lock 19, and your right hand on the left high SEL 1 (on the left inner thigh). (See Figure 4.29.)

2. Place your right hand on the left elbow, at Safety Energy Lock 19, and your left hand on the right high SEL 1 (on the right inner thigh).

SAFETY ENERGY LOCK 15: WASH OUR HEARTS WITH LAUGHTER

Safety Energy Lock 15 is located in the groin. (See Figure 4.30.) By jumper-cabling the SEL 15s, we are better able to restore joy and laughter to our lives, which, of course, changes our perception of everything. Mary refers to the SEL 15s as the "comedians," because they help us take ourselves and situations less seriously.

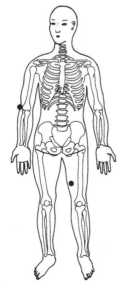

FIGURE 4.29

Safety Energy Lock 15 harmonizes the abdomen, legs, knees, ankles, and feet. It can also be used to aid the heart and alleviate bloat conditions.

To jumper-cable the SEL 15s, place each hand on the left and right groin area and hold. You may also jumper-cable the SEL 15s with the insteps, at SEL 6, followed by the shoulders, at SEL 3. If reaching SEL 6 proves awkward, then SEL 15 may be effectively jumper-cabled with just SEL 3.

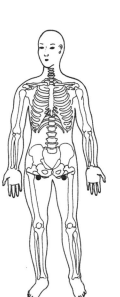

FIGURE 4.30

1. Place your right hand on the right groin, at Safety Energy Lock 15, and your left hand on the right instep, at Safety Energy Lock 6. (See Figure 4.31.) Or place your left hand on the right shoulder, at Safety Energy Lock 3.

2. Place your left hand on the left groin, at Safety Energy Lock 15, and your right hand on the left instep, at Safety Energy Lock 6. Or place your right hand on the left shoulder, at Safety Energy Lock 3.

"A SIXTY-EIGHT-YEAR-OLD MAN was in the hospital following surgery for both femoral arteries, which were totally blocked. The left toes were absolutely black, and the foot was deep purple from a longstanding lack of circulation. The doctors were planning to amputate his

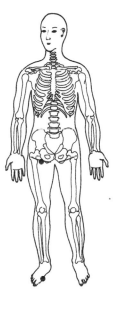

FIGURE 4.31

left leg at the knee as soon as he adequately recovered from the femoral artery surgery.

"I WAS CALLED to the hospital and gave him daily treatments there and at his home when he was released. I used lots of fifteen flows. Each day I could see the color changing. In short, the man did not lose anything, not even a toe. This gentleman continued to receive Jin Shin Jyutsu from me weekly for twelve more years and had a full life, tending his extensive rose garden, bowling, volunteering, and vacationing with his wife and family."

All of the fifteen preceding Safety Energy Locks are contained within the first and second depths. Remember, then, that when we open all of these SELs and keep them free from obstruction, we are also helping to keep the all-important first and second depths in balance.

safety energy locks: 16–26

chapter five

Numbers are keys to the flow of universal energy.

*I*n the last chapter, we explored Safety Energy Locks 1 through 15, located within the first and second depths. Now we will turn our attention to the remaining eleven SELs, which are contained within the third, fourth, and fifth depths.

the third-depth SELs (16–22)

SAFETY ENERGY LOCK 16: TRANSFORMATION

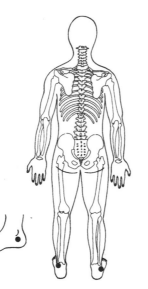

FIGURE 5.1

Safety Energy Lock 16 is located on the outside of the ankle, between the ankle bone and the heel. (See Figure 5.1.) It is opposite Safety Energy Lock 5. When energy flows easily through the SEL 16s, we are better able to make healthy and smooth changes in our lives. For this reason, the SEL 16s are often referred to as "breaking down the old forms and establishing the new."

The SEL 16s harmonize the skeletal system and help improve muscle tone. They are also useful for helping our reproductive functions, aiding elimination, and for relieving head and neck tension.

If holding the SEL 16s is difficult, you can also clear them by utilizing SELs 11 and 25 in the following sequence:

1. Place your right hand on the left shoulder, at Safety Energy Lock 11, and your left hand on the left buttock, at Safety Energy Lock 25. (See Figure 5.2.)

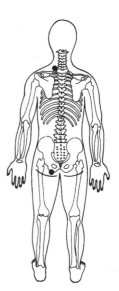

FIGURE 5.2

2. Place your left hand on the right shoulder, at Safety Energy Lock 11, and your right hand on the right buttock, at Safety Energy Lock 25.

"WHEN I WAS a relatively inexperienced practitioner, one of my weekly clients was a woman who had a chronically stiff neck. On one occasion, she arrived at my office visibly shaken. She told me that her husband, an attorney, had lost his job the day before. She was very frightened about the future—the possibility of losing their home, giving up their affluent lifestyle, or even moving away.

"UNCERTAIN AS TO the best way to proceed, my thoughts went to Safety Energy Lock 16. Sixteen breaks down old forms to make room for the new ones. Her old forms certainly seemed to be breaking down. Since I also recalled from my classes that the sixteens help the neck, I decided to treat her by harmonizing that particular SEL. By the end of the hour, the discomfort in her neck had subsided. Her emotional balance also seemed to be restored as she commented to me that she felt more ready to face whatever situation might develop."

SAFETY ENERGY LOCK 17: REPRODUCTIVE ENERGY

Safety Energy Lock 17 is located on the outside of the wrists, on the little-finger side. (See Figure 5.3.) The SEL 17s harmonize the reproductive energy.

The SEL 17s are good to use in emergency situations because they help balance the nervous system. Other areas that benefit when we open them are the heart,

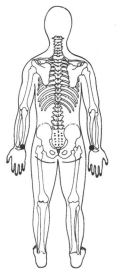

FIGURE 5.3

breast, and ankles. They are also useful for relieving bloat.

To jumper-cable the SEL 17s, simply hold the right wrist with your left hand for several minutes, then the left wrist with your right hand. (See Figure 5.4.)

"AFTER SHE HAD received surgery as an outpatient, I brought my mother home from the hospital. Shortly after helping her into the bathroom, I heard her frantically call me. As I ran in, I saw that she was fainting and falling over. I caught her and began to hold her seventeens. I had often thought, 'Who would remember to do this in an emergency?' whenever I would look at my class notes. Yet at this time I did remember, and she quickly came to."

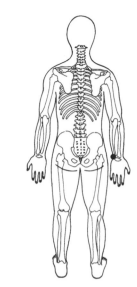

FIGURE 5.4

SAFETY ENERGY LOCK 18: BODY CONSCIOUSNESS AND PERSONALITY

Safety Energy Lock 18 is found on the palm side of the base of the thumb. (See Figure 5.5.) The SEL 18s make us conscious of the physical body and integrate the personality with the physical form.

The SEL 18s harmonize the rib cage and the back of the head. They also assist in eliminating sleep disorders.

To jumper-cable the SEL 18s, hold the base of the right thumb with your left hand for a few minutes. Then apply the same for

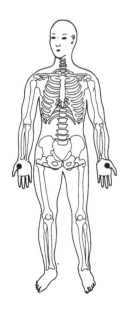

FIGURE 5.5

the other hand: hold the base of the left thumb with your right hand.

Another effective way of clearing the SEL 18s is to jumper-cable SEL 25 and SEL 3, as follows:

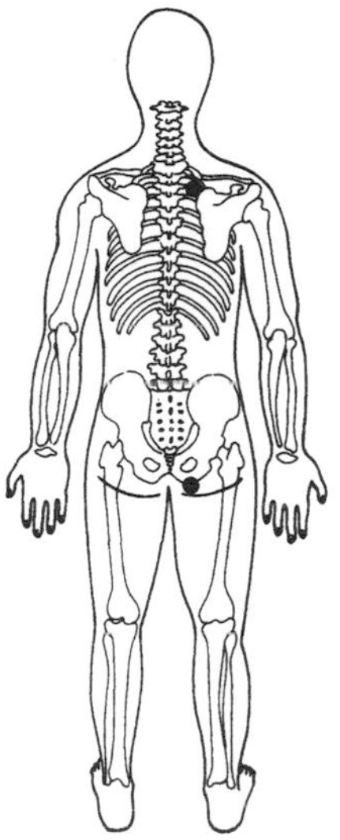

1. Hold the right buttock, at Safety Energy Lock 25, with your right hand, and hold the right shoulder, at Safety Energy Lock 3, with your left hand. (See Figure 5.6.)

2. Jumper-cable the left buttock, at Safety Energy Lock 25, with your left hand, and hold the left shoulder, at Safety Energy Lock 3, with your right hand.

FIGURE 5.6

"WHENEVER I FIND myself at a higher altitude, I seem to be susceptible to headaches. These leave me incapacitated for at least a day. Recently, a friend instructed me on how to hold the base of my thumbs at Safety Energy Lock 18. She told me that this would help to clear up the pressure that I felt in the back of my head. I used this on myself during my next trip to the mountains, and was pleasantly surprised at the result!"

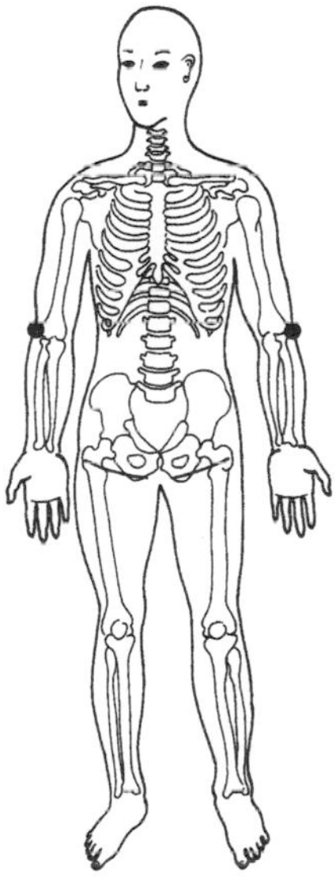

SAFETY ENERGY LOCK 19: PERFECT BALANCE

Safety Energy Lock 19 is found at the crease of the elbows, on the thumb side. (See Figure 5.7.) It is associated with authority,

FIGURE 5.7

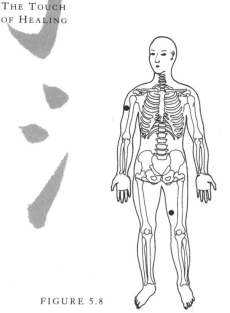

FIGURE 5.8

leadership, and the ability to maintain balance in all kinds of situations. And as we saw earlier, SEL 19 can also be opened when we wish to open Safety Energy Lock 9, which is often difficult to reach.

The SEL 19s harmonize digestion, the back, lungs, and breasts. They also sustain physical fitness and are therefore useful for revitalizing our overall energy.

To jumper-cable the SEL 19s, place your right hand at the thumb-side crease of the left elbow, and your left hand at the crease of the right elbow. To provide an additional outlet for the energy released from the SEL 19s, jumper-cable the high SEL 19s (on the upper arm) while holding the high SEL 1s (on the opposite thigh).

1. Jumper-cable the right upper arm with your left hand, and the left thigh with your right hand. (See Figure 5.8.)

2. Jumper-cable the left upper arm with your right hand, and the right thigh with your left hand.

SAFETY ENERGY LOCK 20: EVERLASTING ETERNITY

Safety Energy Lock 20 is found on the upper part of the forehead, slightly above the eyebrows. (See Figure 5.9.) The SEL 20s unify the personal consciousness with the universal mind and thus allow us to glimpse the timeless reality that we refer to as eternity.

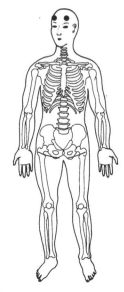

FIGURE 5.9

Opening the SEL 20s harmonizes the ears and eyes. It also helps promote sharper mental activity and restores equilibrium.

To open the SEL 20s, place your left and right hands over the respective safety energy locks and hold them. You may also jumper-cable SEL 22 to release the SEL 20s. The upper-arm-and-thigh sequence recommended for SEL 19 is quite useful for SEL 20 as well.

FIGURE 5.10

1. Jumper-cable the right high SEL 19 (on the upper arm) with your left hand, and the left high SEL 1 (on the thigh) with your right hand. (See Figure 5.10.)

2. Jumper-cable left high SEL 19 (on the upper arm) with your right hand, and the right high SEL 1 (on the thigh) with your left hand.

SAFETY ENERGY LOCK 21: PROFOUND SECURITY AND ESCAPE FROM MENTAL BONDAGE

Safety Energy Lock 21 is found on the underside of the cheekbones, on either side of the face. (See Figure 5.11.) The SEL 21s release the weight of the world, both mentally and physically.

The SEL 21s strengthen thinking, restore energy, and help with balancing weight projects (either overweight or underweight). They are also good for dizziness and stress.

To open the SEL 21s, simply place a hand

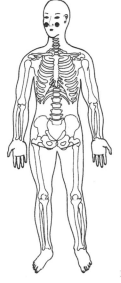

FIGURE 5.11

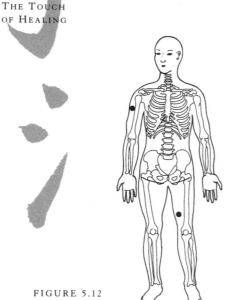

FIGURE 5.12

directly underneath each cheekbone for a few minutes. The exercise suggested for SELs 19 and 20 is also good for releasing any energy stuck in SEL 21.

1. Jumper-cable the right high SEL 19 (on the upper arm) with your left hand, and the left high SEL 1 (on the thigh) with your right hand. (See Figure 5.12.)

2. Jumper-cable the left high SEL 19 (on the upper arm) with your right hand, and the right high SEL 1 (on the thigh) with your left hand.

"A FRIEND OF mine believed that he needed to lose weight in a hurry. Although I have never thought of him as being overweight, I told him that the twenty-ones are good for weight projects. For the next few weeks, he fasted and held the twenty-ones, as I told him to. It's funny— since he really didn't need to lose any weight, he ended up actually gaining a few pounds! The ability of the twenty-ones to correctly balance the body's weight would not allow him to lose any weight."

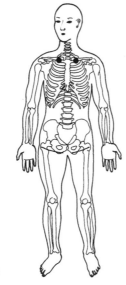

FIGURE 5.13

SAFETY ENERGY LOCK 22: COMPLETE ADAPTATION

Safety Energy Lock 22 is located under the collarbones. (See Figure 5.13.) The SEL 22s are said to balance and harmonize our thoughts because they allow us to think more objectively and reasonably, without emotion or attachment. They also help us to

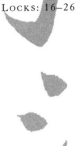

adapt to all new situations and to changes in the environment—including changes in weather or seasons.

Because the SEL 22s represent completion, they are useful for balancing the total being. They also harmonize the thyroid and the parathyroid glands, and they help to prevent strokes. The SEL 22s can be jumper-cabled whenever there is emotional stress or digestive disharmony.

The SEL 22s are jumper-cabled by placing the left and right hands under the collarbones at the site of the safety energy lock and holding that position until the tension melts away. The jumper-cabling sequence used for the previous three SELs is also recommended here.

1. Jumper-cable the right high SEL 19 on the thumb side (on the upper arm) with your left hand, and the left high SEL 1 (on the thigh) with your right hand. (See Figure 5.14.)

2. Jumper-cable the left high SEL 19 (on the upper arm) with your right hand, and the right high SEL 1 (on the thigh) with your left hand.

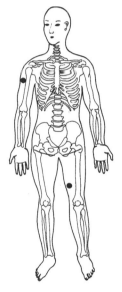

FIGURE 5.14

"I WAS ASKED by Jinny and her husband, Alex, to be present when she gave birth. Jinny was in labor for about fifteen hours before they called me. I arrived at about nine-thirty in the morning and used Jin Shin Jyutsu with her. During that morning I treated her as she lay in bed resting. I worked with her as she walked around the room between contractions, following along beside her. As time went on and on, I could see the look of worry on the nurse's face. She said it was taking too long and whispered in my ear, 'In twenty more minutes

I'm going to recommend the doctor look at her for possible surgery.'

"BY THIS TIME *it was afternoon, and I was searching my brain for a flow that would be most useful. I thought of Mary telling us in class that Safety Energy Lock 22 was excellent for aligning the chest (thirteens), the solar plexus (fourteens), and the groin area (fifteens). I thought, if they are aligned, they are working together in harmony with a good, clear straight pathway for the energy to flow down the front of the body. And if that happens, maybe the energy flowing down will bring the baby with it. So I got behind her, put my hands over her shoulders, and held my right hand under her right collarbone, and my left under her left collarbone. And that's just what happened. On her third exhalation there emerged out into the world a beautiful baby girl, very peacefully, with her eyes open wide in great wonderment."*

the fourth-depth
SEL (23)

Among the first five depths, the fourth depth is unique in that it is the home to just a single safety energy lock, number 23. This unusual circumstance is indicative of the important role of Safety Energy Lock 23. It has a far-reaching influence upon our being. One of the clues to its potency is its location—close by the kidney and adrenal region. The adrenals are the regulators of our "fight-or-flight" response. This, of course, relates to the predominant attitude of the fourth depth—fear. SEL 23, therefore, can be an important tool for helping us eliminate fear.

SAFETY ENERGY LOCK 23: CONTROLLER OF HUMAN DESTINY, PROPER CIRCULATION MAINTENANCE

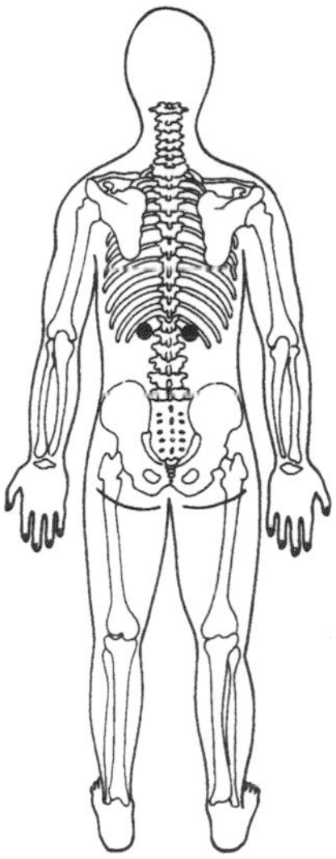

Safety Energy Lock 23 is located in the small of the back. (See Figure 5.15.) The SEL 23s are the controllers of human destiny because they unload fear—an impediment to the natural flow of life.

The SEL 23s improve circulation and adrenal function. They are also good for relieving abdominal distress and reducing temper tantrums. The SEL 23s also help all forms of addiction, projects of the circulatory system, brain function, and physical agility.

FIGURE 5.15

To jumper-cable the SEL 23s, place your left and right hands directly on the small of the back. Hold that position for several minutes, until the tension releases. If that position seems a bit awkward, then open the SEL 23s by jumper-cabling the groin, SEL 15, and the shoulder, SEL 3.

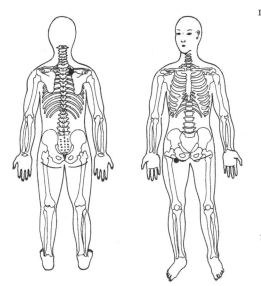

FIGURE 5.16

1. Hold the right groin, at Safety Energy Lock 15, with your right hand, and hold the right shoulder, at Safety Energy Lock 3, with your left hand. (See Figure 5.16.)

2. Hold the left groin, at Safety Energy Lock 15, with your

left hand, and the left shoulder, at Safety Energy Lock 3, with your right hand.

"I WAS STAYING in the hospital with my daughter, Ida, who was admitted in considerable respiratory distress. We had a roommate, Danny, who spent most of his days crying. One day Danny started to moan. His cries sounded even more pained than usual. Soon his bed was surrounded by six or seven staff members. They all stood there discussing which tests to order next as his voice wailed above theirs, 'My stomach! My stomach!' I found myself walking over, and without a word I palmed Danny's twenty-threes. His wails decreased to a whimper, a whisper, then ceased. Danny looked at me right in the eyes, and a slight smile passed over his face. With the crisis apparently over, the staff left the room. One intern and a nurse stayed behind to ask, 'What are you doing?' I explained that by relaxing the back of the waistline, abdominal tensions could be eased.

"THE NEXT DAY, upon entering the room, I found the same nurse sitting in a rocking chair with Danny in her lap, palming his twenty-threes. He was whimpering, but just a little. 'Is this how you do it?' she asked timidly."

the fifth-depth
SELs (24–26)

SAFETY ENERGY LOCK 24: HARMONIZING CHAOS

Safety Energy Lock 24 is found on the outer top of the foot, about midway between the little toe and the ring toe, opposite SEL

6. (See Figure 5.17.) SEL 24 is jumper-cabled whenever we feel confused or chaotic. It promotes peace of mind and body. It is therefore referred to as the "peacemaker."

Appropriately, the SEL 24s are good for eliminating physical manifestations of chaos, such as shakiness. They are also effective for helping us overcome stubbornness, as well as feelings of jealousy and revenge.

The SEL 24s can be jumper-cabled by placing the hands directly upon them. Or they can be jumper-cabled in tandem with the groin.

FIGURE 5.17

1. With your left hand, hold the right outer edge of the shoulder blade, near the armpit, at Safety Energy Lock 26. With your right hand, hold the right groin, at Safety Energy Lock 15. (See Figure 5.18.)

2. With your right hand, hold the left outer edge of the shoulder blade, near the armpit, at Safety Energy Lock 26. With your left hand, hold the left groin, at Safety Energy Lock 15.

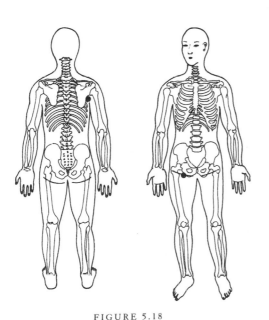

FIGURE 5.18

"I WAS ATTENDING a workshop in Assisi, Italy, last June. A group of about ninety people were traveling on large buses to see the places where Saint Francis had been. The intense meditations and the curvy roads of Tuscany left one member of the group very carsick. She said (in Italian) 'I feel all nauseous and shaky.' I asked the person behind her to hold her twenty-sixes, while I knelt before her and held her twenty-fours. Amazingly, she was fine in about thirty seconds. It was a lot of fun and gratifying to help someone so quickly."

SAFETY ENERGY LOCK 25: QUIETLY REGENERATING

Safety Energy Lock 25, found on the sit-bones (the ischium), is used for calming, soothing, and quietly regenerating all of the body's functions. (See Figure 5.19.)

The SEL 25s increase alertness, energy, and mental clarity.

To jumper-cable them, simply place both hands on the buttocks and hold that position for several minutes. Results may also be achieved by holding SEL 3 along with them, as follows:

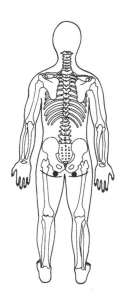

FIGURE 5.19

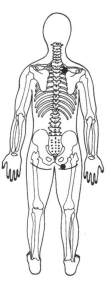

FIGURE 5.20

1. Hold the right buttock, at Safety Energy Lock 25, with your right hand, and hold the right shoulder, at Safety Energy Lock 3, with your left hand. (See Figure 5.20.)

2. Hold the left buttock, at Safety Energy
Lock 25, with your left hand, and hold the
left shoulder, at Safety Energy Lock 3,
with your right hand.

SAFETY ENERGY LOCK 26:
THE DIRECTOR, TOTAL PEACE,
TOTAL HARMONY

Found by the outer edge of the shoulder
blades near the armpit, Safety Energy Lock 26
means "complete." It is opened to provide
harmony and vital life energy to the total being. (See Figure 5.21.)

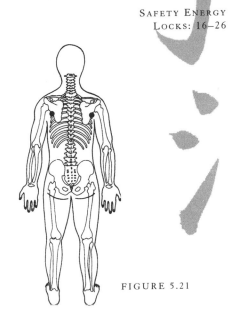

FIGURE 5.21

The SEL 26s recharge all mental and physical functions with vital life energy.

Just quietly fold the arms across the chest, and hold Safety Energy Lock 26. It is okay to hold one at a time or both together. The
following exercise is also a powerful way to
clear SEL 26:

1. Hold the right thumb, index finger,
   middle finger, ring finger, and little
   finger with your left hand, one by one.
   (See Figure 5.22.)

2. Hold the left thumb, index finger, middle
   finger, ring finger, and little finger with
   your right hand, one by one.

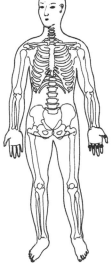

FIGURE 5.22

The importance of the safety energy locks
cannot be overemphasized. As you grow

more familiar with their location, more aware of their purpose, and more comfortable in jumper-cabling them, you will gain a corresponding sense of confidence in your ability to deal with almost any conceivable disharmony.

Each of the twenty-six safety energy locks represents a site of highly concentrated energy. Mostly, our discussion of them has focused on their role as circuit-breakers. Yet they are also places of high conductivity, energetic junctures along the Supervisor Flows for much of the body's various other flows. In the next chapter we will take a closer look at these various flows—known in Jin Shin Jyutsu as the twelve organ flows.

the organ flows

chapter six

The harmonizing mechanics
for the elements.

As we have come to learn, flows are like rivers of energy that run through each of us. When these rivers are clear of obstruction, energy moves freely throughout the body. Yet when the river becomes too tumultuous or constricted, the movement of energy is disrupted. Eddies form, and the energy spills over its banks. Certain areas become unnecessarily flooded, thereby depriving other regions of their fundamental energy needs.

In Chapter 3 we set about familiarizing ourselves with the three primary energy rivers within us, the Trinity Flows. These were the Main Central Flow and the left and right Supervisor Flows. Along with these three primary flows, there are twelve additional flows that also play a vital role in distributing life energy to all parts of our being. In this chapter we will focus our attention upon these twelve flows, which are known as the organ flows.

During the course of his studies, Jiro Murai noted that a unique relationship exists between each of these twelve flows and a particular organ. Although each flow is known by the name of its related organ, such as the liver flow or the gall bladder flow, the entire flow and its respective organ form an integrated and singular whole. The flow is not separate from the organ. On the contrary, the organ is the most condensed manifestation of the flow. For this reason, the proper name of each flow includes the words *function energy,* so that, say, the lung flow is known as the *Lung Function Energy.* Thus the name is representative of the entire flow, not just of the organ.

Each flow has its own distinct route through the body. At its completion the energy within that flow moves on to become another flow, rather than merely stopping. For example, after the life energy runs through the liver flow, it moves on and becomes the lung flow; from the lung flow, the energy continues on to become the large intestine flow. Thus, a continual movement of energy is maintained within the body. All twelve organ flows collectively create a single, unified circuit of energy that is constantly running throughout the entire body. The harmony or disharmony of these twelve flows is studied by Jin Shin Jyutsu practitioners by "listening" to the twelve pulses on the wrists (six on each). (A discussion of these pulses is beyond the scope of this book but is extensively elaborated upon in Jin Shin Jyutsu classes.)

the route
to harmony

Blockage in the flows can also be detected by the appearance of certain disharmonies. A disruption within a particular flow can manifest itself as a symptom anywhere along its pathway. As we shall soon see, the flows are often quite long and intricate, which means that a disharmony can occur far from its associated organ. For example, the Spleen Function Energy ascends from the inner side of the big toenail, up through the leg, and into the abdomen. From there, the energy flow travels to the spleen, where it divides into two separate branches. One branch ends its journey at the root of the tongue, where the energy scatters, while the other ascends to the center of the chest and flows into the heart. (See Figure 6.7.)

We can see from this example that the spleen flow is essential to the health and vitality of an enormous part of the body. An imbalance in the spleen flow can appear as a disharmony anywhere along the flow. This applies to all the other flows as well. By knowing the flow routes, we can understand the underlying cause of a symptom and how it can be harmonized. We can then use the appropriate Jin Shin Jyutsu sequences to restore balance to the flow.

Each of the individual organ flows not only provides life energy but resonates with a particular aspect of our consciousness. Thus the manner by which energy travels along these unique pathways affects both our physical body and our mental and emotional being. Similarly, each of the twelve organ flows can be unfavorably influenced by any of the attitudes (discussed in Chapter 2). The stomach and spleen flows, for example, are adversely affected by worry and anxiety. Conversely, people who have a deep optimism and a large capacity for understanding are better able to maintain harmony within the stomach and spleen flows.

Jin Shin Jyutsu, as we have frequently noted, enables us to develop an awareness of the interrelationship of the various aspects of our being. Along these lines, an awareness of the twelve organ flows helps provide us with a deep and very specific understanding of our innate biorhythms. Each of these flows receives its most abundant supply of energy during a specific two-hour period of the day. Similarly, related pairs of flows receive their most abundant life energy during a particular season. Sometimes when an organ flow is in disharmony, we may experience some physical, mental, or emotional symptom—such as fatigue, the loss of clarity, or the arousal of a particular attitude. However, when we are aware of the hours that an organ flow is receiving optimal energy, we receive additional insight into both the source of a particular imbalance and the means by which we are best able to restore harmony.

Finally, since each of the twelve organ flows arises out of a particular depth, we can keep them balanced by simply holding a particular finger. Or, as we are about to see, we might also balance a particular flow by jumper-cabling two safety energy locks that are located along it.

the twelve organ flows

What follows is a description of the pathway of each organ flow. Because some of these flows are rather elaborate, we have illustrated them for reference. In addition, each flow description includes the time of day and the season in which it is most imbued with energy; the attitude that is associated with its disharmony; and the finger and safety energy locks that can help us harmonize it. Keep in mind, as you read these descriptions, that each function energy is composed of a left and right flow, which are mirror images of each other.

Also, please note that occasionally a discrepancy exists between the written description and the illustrations of particular energy pathways. This is especially evident as we trace their route along the arms. To avoid unnecessary confusion, bear in mind that the original reference point for these diagrams is a standing body with arms extended above the head, palms facing outward with the thumbs toward the mid-line of the body.

Therefore, upward or ascending notes the movement of energy from the shoulder to the fingers while descending refers to the movement of energy from the fingers to the shoulders.

LUNG FUNCTION ENERGY

> From the lungs the record
>
> of man's every thought,
>
> word, and deed passes
>
> into the blood to be
>
> carried to seed.

The Lung Function Energy arises from the Liver Function Energy in the stomach, beginning at four A.M. (See Figure 6.1.)

In the stomach, the lung energy intermingles with digested food juices, then divides itself in two. The smaller of the two flows is sent to the outer surface of the large intestine (not il-

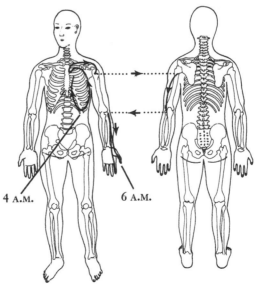

4 A.M.   6 A.M.

FIGURE 6.1

lustrated). The larger flow circulates through the diaphragm and then travels into the lung area.

This larger energy flow circulates throughout the lungs and gathers in the trachea. From there, it flows to the projection at the outside of the shoulder blade (known as the acromion). From the acromion, it travels to where the front part of the shoulder joins with the arm. It then moves to the underarm and along the outer side of the arm.

After moving along to the front side of the arm, the lung flow progresses to the outer side of the elbow. From there, it advances to an area about five inches below the wrist. Here again the energy separates into two distinct flows. The smaller of these flows moves to the inner side of the thumbnail, where it circulates the nail before enveloping the thumb. The other, larger flow goes to the inner side of the index fingernail, where it changes into the Large Intestine Function Energy. (See Figure 6.3.)

The Lung Function Energy takes two hours to complete its circulating pattern. Its peak energy hours are between four and six A.M. At six, the Lung Function Energy becomes the Large Intestine Function Energy.

The season during which the lung flow receives its optimal amount of energy is autumn.

The attitude associated with lung flow disharmony is sadness.

Balancing the Lung Flow

The lung flow arises out of the second depth. As we saw in Chapter 2, the second depth is balanced by jumper-cabling the ring finger. To balance and harmonize the lung flow, hold each ring finger.

Here is a "quickie" method to balance the Lung Function Energy, using the safety energy locks:

1. Place your left hand on the left SEL 14 (at the front bottom of the rib cage). At the same time, place your right hand on the left SEL 22 (under the collarbone). (See Figure 6.2.)

2. Place your right hand on the right SEL
14 (at the front bottom of the rib cage).
At the same time, place your left hand on
the right SEL 22 (under the collarbone).

*"PETE WAS A postal worker who had taken
disability leave because of an asthmatic
condition. He used an oxygen tank, could
no longer walk any distance, and could not
drive his car.*

*"AFTER HIS FIRST Jin Shin Jyutsu session,
when he received a lung flow, he was able
to walk around the block. Two weeks
later, he went to the desert with his family,*
*which was at least a 150-mile trip along a two-lane road that
wound through the mountains. He drove the entire round
trip!"*

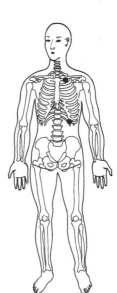

FIGURE 6.2

LARGE INTESTINE
FUNCTION ENERGY

Both the mind and

the bowels need to

be open.

Starting from the index
finger, the Large Intes-
tine Function Energy
flows up the back side of
the arm. (See Figure
6.3.) It moves along the
front of the shoulder,

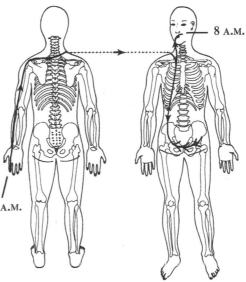

FIGURE 6.3

then passes through the first thoracic vertebra, located at the top of the back. At that point, the energies from the left and right flows (remember, they are mirror images of each other, on each side of the body) meet and briefly intermingle.

After its rendezvous with the right flow, the left flow moves around the right side of the neck and down into the right chest. It rises from there up into the right breast, where it separates into two parts.

One part circulates the right lung, then moves down the diaphragm to a point very close to the navel. There, the energy describes a half-circle before scattering at the outer area of the large intestine.

The second part flows from the right breast up through the right side of the throat into the right lower gums. It goes on to circulate along the right side of the face before making its way between the nose and upper lip. From there, it flows over to the left cheekbone, where it becomes the Stomach Function Energy.

From the top of the spine, the right flow travels in an identical path along the opposite side of the body. Both the left and right large intestine flows take two hours to complete their route. The flows' peak hours occur between six and eight A.M.

The season during which the large intestine flow receives the optimal amount of energy is the autumn.

The attitude associated with large intestine flow disharmony is sadness, or grief.

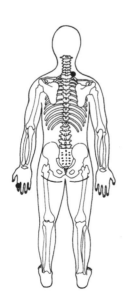

FIGURE 6.4

Balancing the Large Intestine Flow

Since the large intestine flow is born of the second depth, you can harmonize it yourself by holding your ring finger. Or you may help another person harmonize theirs by using the following "quickie" sequence:

1. Place your left hand on the right SEL 11 (at the upper back, below where the neck meets the shoulders). At the same time, hold your left index finger with the right hand. (See Figure 6.4.)

2. Place your right hand on the left SEL 11 (at the upper back, below where the neck meets the shoulders). At the same time, hold your right index finger with the left hand.

> "*WHEN MY DAUGHTER Danielle was about four or five years old, I enrolled her in ballet class. Running across the waxed gym floor, my little girl fell face-first, banging her baby tooth into the hard floor. One hour later my sweetheart came home and burst into tears. The whole upper lip was swollen and bleeding. The trauma to the tooth had forced it up into the gum, possibly damaging her permanent front tooth. The inside of her lip had a gash where the tooth had pierced it. I held her, cupping my right hand over her lip and placing my left hand on top of my right. I didn't touch the area because it was so painful. When she said it felt better, I sang to her to distract her and gave the area some extra jumper-cabling. The swelling reduced, the abrasion disappeared, and the color was normal.*
>
> "*THAT NIGHT AS she slept, I used a large intestine flow because it relates to the jaws and gums.*
>
> "*IN THE MORNING I was asked why I hadn't visited the dentist immediately, as a permanent front tooth requires prompt attention. In fact, when I reached the dentist's office, he was amazed. He wanted to know what had happened to the hematoma and how we had closed the wound so fast.*
>
> "*AFTER VIEWING THE X ray, he felt we should pull the baby tooth as a precaution. He also advised me that the blood that had collected in the area of the permanent front tooth would cause it to blacken.*

"WE DIDN'T PULL any teeth. We continued helping the large intestine flow over the years, and now, at fourteen, my daughter has the whitest, most beautiful front teeth."

STOMACH FUNCTION ENERGY

Stomach function

represents reason and

intelligence.

After changing over from the Large Intestine Function Energy at the cheekbone at 8:00 A.M., the Stomach Function Energy flows up to a point centered between the eyebrows. (See Figure 6.5.) Here both the left- and right-side flows meet before going their separate ways.

The left flow continues on to an area underneath the right eye. From there, it descends along the jawline, back toward a spot just above the eyebrow—in front of the left ear. At that point, the energy turns toward the eyes and descends to the left side acromion (outer shoulder blade). At the acromion, the flow separates into two parts, which we will refer to as A and B.

Part A flows inward and goes directly into the stomach, where it further divides itself into parts 1 and 2. Part 1 flows into the umbilicus (or navel). From the umbilicus, it crosses over to the right thigh. As it travels along the inner thigh toward the outside of the knee, it meets up with the B flow en route. The left 2, after leaving the stomach, flows through the gall bladder, the right kidney, and finally into the twelfth thoracic vertebra, where it scatters. (On the other side, the right 2 moves through the spleen and left kidney, before scattering at the twelfth thoracic vertebra.)

On its way down from the acromion, the left B flow travels into the abdomen. About one inch to the left of the navel (umbilicus), it flows into the groin, where it intermingles with the 1. From there, it descends the inner side of the right thigh, to a point about three inches above the knee. It then continues diagonally through the knee. At the outer side of the knee, B separates into parts 3 and 4.

Part 3 descends along the outer side of the right leg into the middle toe. Part 4 descends into the top of the instep and separates into two parts. One part of 4 travels to the index toe. The second part flows into the outer side of the big toe, where it becomes the Spleen Function Energy.

Except for the route taken by its 2 branch, the right-side stomach flow travels a similar path along the opposite side of the body. The peak time for both the left and right flows is between eight and ten A.M. At ten A.M., the Stomach Function Energy becomes the Spleen Function Energy.

The season during which the stomach flow receives the optimal amount of energy is the hottest part of summer.

The attitude associated with disharmony of the stomach flow is worry.

Balancing the Stomach Flow

The stomach flow arises from the first depth. Thus all you need to do to balance it is simply to hold the thumb of each hand for a few minutes apiece. You can also open SEL 21 and SEL 22, as follows:

1. Place your right hand on the left SEL 21 (at the underside of the

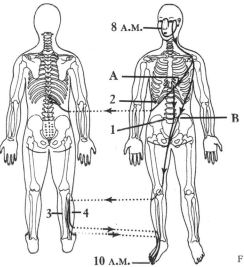

FIGURE 6.5

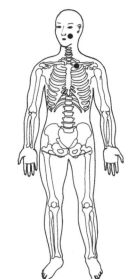

FIGURE 6.6

cheekbone). At the same time, jumper-cable the left SEL 22 (under the collarbone) with your left hand. (See Figure 6.6.)

2. Place your left hand on the right SEL 21 (at the underside of the cheekbone). At the same time, jumper-cable the right SEL 22 (under the collarbone) with your right hand.

"MAT, MY OLDEST son, was assaulted. The police caught the offender, and Mat was taken to the hospital, where it was deter-mined by X rays that he suffered a fractured jaw and needed surgery that afternoon. Mat's first phone call was to me, asking for Jin Shin Jyutsu. I arrived at the hospital at about eleven A.M. and started what amounted to about six hours of jumper-cabling, using mainly the stomach flow. Meanwhile, the doctor postponed surgery until the following day, as she wanted to confer with another doctor. She came in at three P.M. to examine Mat and found him improved. I left for home at six-thirty P.M. When I arrived, there was a message from the doctor saying she had been to see Mat again and sent him home as he no longer required surgery! What a gift!"

SPLEEN FUNCTION ENERGY

Gateway for solar energy.

From the big toe (where it took over from the Stomach Function Energy) at ten A.M., the Spleen Function Energy ascends toward the inner ankle, through the heel, and up the inner leg. (See Figure 6.7.) At the back of the knee, the flow advances up the inner leg to the groin, where it crosses over to the abdomen on the opposite side. From there the energy continues its ascent up to the ninth rib. There the flow separates into two parts, A and B.

Part A goes up to the third rib, then turns toward the underarm before descending back down toward the seventh rib. At the seventh rib A turns outward toward the back, where it begins an ascent toward the throat. A then passes through the throat to the root of the tongue, where the energy scatters.

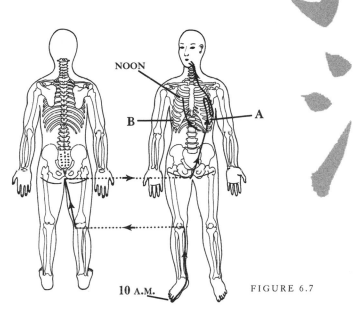

FIGURE 6.7

Part B, meanwhile, has circulated the outer surface of the stomach, then ascended up the center of the chest into the heart, where it becomes the Heart Function Energy.

The peak hours for the spleen flow are between ten o'clock and twelve noon. At noon, the Spleen Function Energy becomes the Heart Function Energy. Like the stomach flow, it receives its optimal amount of energy during the hottest part of summer.

The attitude associated with spleen flow disharmony is worry.

To Balance the Spleen Flow

The spleen flow arises out of the first depth. To balance the spleen flow and the first depth, hold the thumb.

The following "quickie" sequence is recommended for balancing the spleen flow:

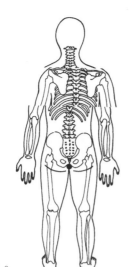

FIGURE 6.8

1. Place your right hand on the right SEL 5 (between the ankle bone and the heel). At the same time, place your left hand on the coccyx. (See Figure 6.8.)

2. Place your left hand on the left SEL 5 (between the ankle bone and the heel). At the same time, place your right hand on the coccyx.

"I WAS TRAVELING in Oaxaca, Mexico, with a girlfriend in 1980 and ingested some bad food or water. I became really ill, with nausea, fever, and weakness. I instructed my friend to use a spleen flow for me, as I was too weak to apply it myself.

"BY THE FOLLOWING morning, my symptoms were cleared and I was ready to continue traveling. This really showed me how profound Jin Shin Jyutsu can be in acute situations. We met several people along our journey who had gotten food poisoning and were laid up for three to six days."

HEART FUNCTION ENERGY

> The body is in the heart,
>
> as the oak is in the acorn.

At noon, after the Spleen Function Energy has changed over to the Heart Function Energy, it splits into five separate branches—A, B, C, D, and E. All flow out the four exits of the heart. (See Figure 6.9.)

Part A flows through the third thoracic vertebra and then out to the chest.

Part B descends through the underarm region toward the back. Passing through the seventh thoracic vertebra, the left-side B flows to the right kidney, while the right-side B flows into the left kidney.

Part C descends from the lower exit of the heart, through the diaphragm, to an area about one inch above the umbilicus. From there, C flows into the small intestine.

From the third front rib, part D ascends up into the throat, after which it passes through the eyes and into the cerebrum.

Part E ascends through the chest. The left side of the E branch travels into the left lung; the right side into the right lung. From there, both the left and right side branches of E circulate through the trachea before proceeding along to the underarm on its respective side. From the underarm, the left E travels into the left arm; the right E branch into the right arm. There, the energy advances along the front part of each arm and through the elbow until it reaches the inner side of the nail of the little finger. This is the point at which the Heart Function Energy becomes the Small Intestine Function Energy.

The daily peak time for the heart flow is from noon to two P.M. The season in which heart energy peaks is summer.

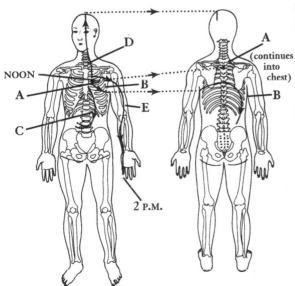

FIGURE 6.9

Pretense (or trying-to) is the attitude associated with a disharmony in the heart flow.

To Balance the Heart Flow

The heart flow arises out of the fifth depth. Accordingly, you can harmonize it by balancing the fifth depth. You can facilitate this by holding either one of your little fingers.

The following easy-to-use "quickie" is also recommended for the Heart Function Energy:

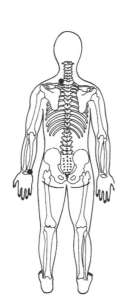

FIGURE 6.10

1. Place your left hand on the left SEL 11 (at the upper back, below where the neck meets the shoulders). At the same time, place your right hand on the left SEL 17 (on the outside of the wrists, toward the little-finger side of the wrist). (See Figure 6.10.)

2. Place your right hand on the right SEL 11 (at the upper back, below where the neck meets the shoulders). At the same time, place your left hand on the right SEL 17 (on the outside of the wrists, toward the little-finger side of the wrist).

"MY MOM HAD a heart attack this past February, and my dad had one exactly a year before Mom's. Anyway, she would hear me tell my dad to hold his little finger. Well, this is practically one of the only things my mom knows about Jin Shin Jyutsu, but she held on to her little finger all the way to the hospital, and we know that her little finger saved her life. The doctors

*told my sister-in-law, who is the head nurse of the ICU, that
according to the EKG, my mom should have had a massive
heart attack—the Big One, they called it. She didn't! I arrived
at the hospital that night and jumper-cabled, then again the
next morning and night. The next day they went in expecting
to find a major blockage in the left ventricle. There was just a
tiny blockage. WOW! Actually, same thing with my dad—I
had jumper-cabled him three times before his stress test—to
see how much damage was done to the heart. The doctor said
he could not believe it, but there were no signs of a heart
attack. Needless to say, my mom and dad love their little
fingers and hold them daily."*

SMALL INTESTINE FUNCTION ENERGY

The vehicle of illumination.

At two P.M., from the inner side
of the little fingernail, the
Small Intestine Function
Energy descends to the
outer side of the little fingernail, the outer side of
the elbow, and up
through the back of the
shoulder. (See Figure
6.11.)

At the top of the back,
left and right energy in-
termingle at the first thoracic vertebra. From there,
the left small intestine flow

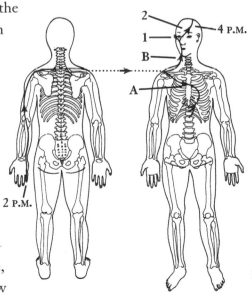

FIGURE 6.11

moves around the right side of the neck and down into the right shoulder at the front of the arm joint. There, it separates into two parts, A and B.

Part A flows into the breast, then moves diagonally into the heart. From there, it flows into the stomach and scatters.

Part B ascends into the right cheekbone and separates into two parts, 1 and 2. Part 1 flows under the right eye and into the right ear. Part 2 ascends to the forehead, above the center of the left eyebrow, where it becomes the Bladder Function Energy at four P.M.

The right flow follows an identical path, along the opposite side of the body. The Small Intestine Function Energy's peak hours are between two and four P.M. The season in which the small intestine flow receives the greatest amount of energy is summer.

The attitude of pretense, or trying-to, is associated with disharmony in the small intestine flow.

To Balance the Small Intestine Flow

The fifth depth gives rise to the small intestine flow. To balance the fifth depth and small intestine, jumper-cable the little finger on both hands. Or use the following sequence of SELs:

1. Place your left hand on the left SEL 11 (at the upper back, below where the neck meets the shoulders). At the

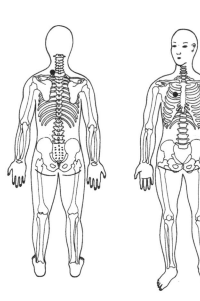

FIGURE 6.12

same time, place your right hand on the right SEL 13 (at the front of the rib cage, by the third rib). (See Figure 6.12.)

2. Place your right hand on the right SEL 11 (at the upper back, below where the neck meets the shoulders). At the same time, place your left hand on the left SEL 13 (at the front of the rib cage, by the third rib).

"MY SON, SASHA, age 16, is a professional clown at children's birthday parties. He does a thirty-minute magic show in front of ten to forty people, then paints the children's faces and makes them balloon animals.

"HE BEGAN WHEN he was just fourteen. He would get quite nervous a few days before the party. He was a teenager doing a job that adults usually do, and I'm sure that put added pressure on him.

"BECAUSE HE WAS 'pre-tense,' as Mary says—tense before the actual event—I focused on the fifth depth and used a small intestine flow for him several times. We forgot about it, but on Sunday after the party he said, 'Wow! Mom, that was the first time I didn't get nervous before a clown gig. That was great.'"

BLADDER FUNCTION ENERGY

Takes away our tears and fears.

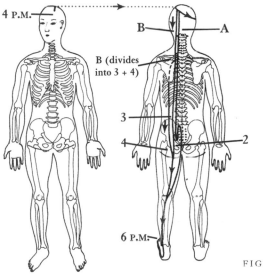

FIGURE 6.13

At four P.M., from the forehead, the Bladder Function Energy ascends diagonally to the center of the top of the head. (See Figure 6.13.) There, the left- and right-side bladder flows briefly cross paths. Shortly after they resume their separate courses, both flows divide themselves into two parts. One of these parts flows into the earlobe and scatters. The other part flows into the brain area. As it emerges from the brain, it once again divides into two distinct parts, A and B.

Traveling about one inch to the side of the spinal column, part A descends into the coccyx. From there, it flows into the bladder and, as it moves inward and up, separates into two parts, 1 and 2.

Part 1 ascends into the kidney, then descends into the bladder, after which it ascends again (not illustrated).

Part 2 follows the hipbone and emerges to the side of the coccyx, behind the rectum. From there, it descends to the back of the knee and intermingles with part 4, described below.

Meanwhile, after separating from part A, part B travels to the back of the shoulder, where it separates into two parts (3 and 4).

Part 3 descends, following a route about one and a half inches to the side of the spinal column, to the ischium (the sit-bone).

Part 4 also descends along a path about three inches out from the spinal column. It, too, finds its way to the ischium, where it intermingles with 3. From the ischium, 4 descends to the back of the knee and intermingles with 2. It then continues its descent along the outer side of the leg, eventually passing through the ankle to the outer side of the little toe. At the little toe, part 4 of the Bladder Function Energy becomes the Kidney Function Energy.

The peak hours of the Bladder Function

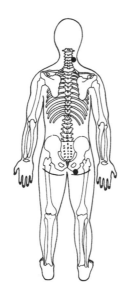

FIGURE 6.14

Energy are four to six P.M. The bladder flow receives the most abundant energy in the winter.

The attitude associated with disharmony of the bladder flow is fear (*F*alse *E*vidence *A*ppearing *R*eal).

To Balance the Bladder Flow

The bladder flow is associated with the fourth depth and is harmonized either by holding the index fingers of both hands or by utilizing the following "quickie" sequence:

1. Place your left hand on the right SEL 12 (at the back of neck, midway between the skull and the shoulders). At the same time, use your right hand to jumper-cable the right SEL 25 (at the ischium). (See Figure 6.14.)

2. Place your right hand on the left SEL 12 (at the back of neck, midway between the skull and the shoulders). At the same time, use your left hand to jumper-cable the left SEL 25 (at the ischium).

> "*AN ACQUAINTANCE OF mine called to tell me that she had finally convinced her son and daughter-in-law to bring their eight-month-old son to see me. He was scheduled for surgery because his tear duct was closed. She knew they were humoring her, but she asked me to please do something because she couldn't bear to see such a young baby have surgery. This was when I was just a beginning student.*
>
> "*I ANXIOUSLY PULLED out my books to see what flow I would use. There in the first line of the bladder flow explanation page was 'closed tear duct.' This little active eight-month-old was quite a challenge, but I managed to use the bladder flow. After the second session the mother called and said that the surgery was canceled because the duct had opened.*"

KIDNEY FUNCTION ENERGY

The life essence for

individual development.

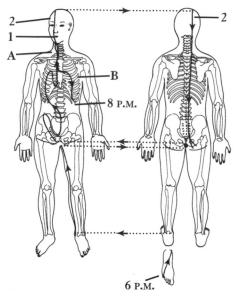

FIGURE 6.15

At six P.M., from the outer side of the little toe, the Kidney Function Energy flows diagonally across the sole of the foot. (See Figure 6.15.) Traveling underneath the inner heel, it turns up the inner part of the leg and goes through the inner groin and on to the rectum.

From the rectum, the flow crosses over to the opposite side of the coccyx, after which it travels from the back to the front of the reproductive organ. Continuing onward, the energy moves along the pubic bone into the lower abdomen and then on to the umbilicus. Upon leaving the umbilicus, it proceeds to the kidney. The left-side kidney flow goes to the right kidney, while the right-side flow travels to the left kidney.

From either kidney, the flow descends into the bladder, after which it ascends to the eighth rib and into the liver. After passing through the liver, it flows into the lower end of the stomach (pylorus), up to the fourth rib and into the lung, where it separates into two parts, A and B.

Part A ascends through the throat until it reaches the root of the tongue, where it further separates into two parts, 1 and 2. Part 1 scatters at the root of the tongue. Part 2 ascends along the side of the nose and up the forehead, before descending the back of the

head. It then continues its downward flow, following a path about one-half inch to the side of the spinal column. Eventually, part 2 emerges at the front of the groin, where it scatters.

Part B moves from the lung to the third front rib and into the heart. The energy passes through the lower part of the heart and into the diaphragm, where it becomes the Diaphragm Function Energy.

The Kidney Function Energy is at its peak from six to eight P.M. The season during which it receives the optimal energy is the winter.

The attitude associated with kidney flow disharmony is fear.

To Balance the Kidney Flow

The kidney flow arises out of the fourth depth. Therefore, jumper-cabling the index finger and balancing the fourth depth help balance the kidney flow.

This "quickie" also enables us to directly harmonize the kidney flow:

1. Hold the left little toe with your right hand. Place your left hand upon the pubic bone. (See Figure 6.16.)

2. Hold the right little toe with your left hand. Place your right hand upon the pubic bone.

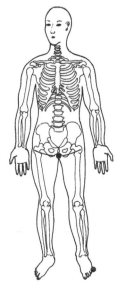

FIGURE 6.16

"MY ROOMMATE'S ESOPHAGUS periodically became constricted. As a boy, Randy had swallowed a caustic solution. Although he vomited almost immediately, the solution caused his esophagus to contract to a small opening—even aspirin had to be chewed well rather than swallowed whole. Randy

*told me that every five years or so his esophagus closed
completely. One day this began to occur. He didn't want to go
to the hospital for help, as the solution for opening his
esophagus was to 'ram' a flexible tube filled with medication
through the passage. Instead he asked me for Jin Shin Jyutsu.
I used a kidney flow because I read in one of the texts that
disharmony may result in 'swelling developing at the top of
the esophagus.' We were both relieved when Randy got up
after receiving Jin Shin Jyutsu, went to the sink to get a glass
of water, and drank. His esophagus no longer felt constricted!"*

DIAPHRAGM FUNCTION ENERGY

The source of life itself.

At eight P.M. the Diaphragm Function Energy flows out of the diaphragm and into the heart. (See Figure 6.17.) Leaving the heart,
it travels behind the third rib, where it separates into two parts, A
and B.

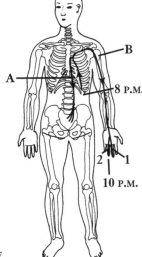

Part A descends and circulates the stomach before continuing its descent to an area
about an inch below the umbilicus. There it
scatters into the small intestine.

Part B emerges from the third rib, to the
side of the breast. From there, it moves under the arm, then ascends the front of the
arm. From there, it follows a path from the
outer elbow to the center front of the elbow,
before continuing on to the center of the
palm. There it separates into two parts, 1
and 2.

Part 1 flows to the tip of the middle finger. Part 2 flows to the inner side of the ring

FIGURE 6.17

finger and circulates the tip of the nail before changing over to the Umbilicus Function Energy.

The peak hours for the Diaphragm Function Energy are from eight to ten P.M. Because the diaphragm is contained within the sixth depth (totality), its associated season is year-round.

Total despondency is associated with a disharmony of the diaphragm flow.

To Balance the Diaphragm Flow

The diaphragm arises out of the sixth depth. To harmonize the sixth depth and the diaphragm, jumper-cable the palm of the hand. The following sequence is also an effective tool for balancing this flow:

1. Place your right hand on the left SEL 14 (at the front bottom of the rib cage). Hold the right SEL 19 (at the elbow crease, on the thumb side) with your left hand. (See Figure 6.18.)

2. Place your left hand on the right SEL 14 (at the front bottom of the rib cage). Hold the left SEL 19 (at the elbow crease, on the thumb side) with your right hand.

"MY SISTERS AND I were born in the 1940s in the Pioneer Valley in western Massachusetts. Our summer evenings were spent watching airplanes swooping down, dusting tobacco fields with DDT. The effects of the poison on our bodies were both immediate and long-term. One of the many long-term effects was that our growing arms and legs bent out of shape. When Mom asked our family doctor why her children were deforming, Dr. Clark

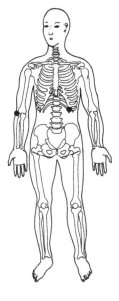

FIGURE 6.18

said, 'It's all the children in the valley. The cause is environmental.'

"BY MY MID-TWENTIES, every aspect of my being was weak: breathing, assimilation, elimination, immune system, eyesight. I had become hyperactive and felt mentally and emotionally stuck.

"IN 1981 I started studying Jin Shin Jyutsu with Mary. With her able guidance and my increasing awareness and understanding, I am able to use my jumper cables to energize my total being by utilizing my Diaphragm and Umbilicus Function Energy. They help my sixth depth, which represents 'the expanding principle of motion'—just what I needed to reverse the contraction my body was experiencing. By energizing my Diaphragm Function Energy, I watched my slanted eyes straighten, my flushed face lighten, my accelerated pulse quiet, my breathing improve, and all my body functions stabilize.

"NOW, WHEN MY total being gets discombobulated by something, I hold my palm or use the diaphragm flow 'quickie' to receive the energy I need, and I feel myself return to balance." (This story continues at the end of the Umbilicus Function Energy section.)

UMBILICUS FUNCTION ENERGY

Guardian of all the organs.

At ten P.M., after taking over from the Diaphragm Function Energy at the outer ring fingernail, the Umbilicus Function Energy ascends the back of the wrist. (See Figure 6.19.) Flowing by the elbow and the joint of the arm and shoulder, the energy arrives at the third front rib (between the breasts), where it separates into two parts, A and B.

Part A initially scatters at a point opposite the third rib cartilage. It then continues flowing through the fifth rib before traveling into the heart. From the heart, the left side of A passes through the pancreas and into the stomach. The right side of A delivers energy to the gall bladder before it, too, enters the stomach.

Part B (on both the left and right sides) ascends to the shoulder and passes through the neck muscle and the first thoracic vertebra, to a point about two inches from the opposite ear. At the ear, B divides into parts 1 and 2.

Part 1 moves from the back of the ear, diagonally through the head, and emerges at the inner edge of the eyebrow. From there, it crosses to the outer edge of the eye and into the occipital bone, where the left and right flow intermingle.

In the meantime, part 2 flows from the back of the ear into the ear itself, before traveling out to the center of the lower eyelid. At this point, part 2 of the Umbilicus Function Energy becomes the Gall Bladder Function Energy.

The hours during which the Umbilicus Function Energy receives the maximum energy are between ten P.M. and midnight. Its associated season is also year-round.

Like the diaphragm flow, a disharmony of the umbilicus flow can result in total despondency.

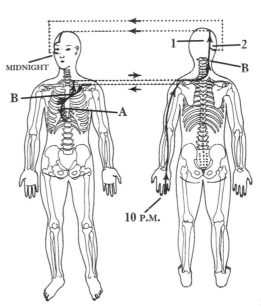

FIGURE 6.19

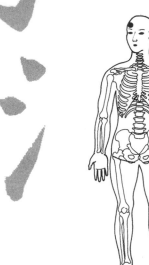

FIGURE 6.20

To Balance the Umbilicus Flow

The umbilicus flow arises out of the sixth depth and is therefore harmonized by jumper-cabling the palm. The "quickies" are the SEL 19s and the SEL 20s.

1. Place your left hand on the right SEL 20 (at the upper part of the forehead, slightly above the eyebrows). At the same time use your right hand to jumper-cable the left SEL 19 (at the elbow crease, on the thumb side). (See Figure 6.20.)

2. Place your right hand on the left SEL 20 (at the upper part of the forehead, slightly above the eyebrows). At the same time use your left hand to jumper-cable the right SEL 19 (at the elbow crease, on the thumb side).

(THIS STORY IS continued from the Diaphragm Energy Function section.) "By energizing my Umbilicus Function Energy, all the weaknesses I've experienced have improved; many have disappeared. The Umbilicus Function Energy has truly gotten my body into order. I am really enjoying my straight limbs and erect spine, improved assimilation, elimination, stamina, eyesight, resistance to viruses, and calm.

"SINCE MY FORTY-FIFTH year, I'm experiencing changes in my menstrual cycle. My body's ability to handle the smooth flow of bodily substances, a function of the umbilicus flow, is put to the test on a monthly basis. When I experience symptoms like headaches, neck tension, ear ringing, night sweats, or bloat, I utilize the Umbilicus Function Energy and watch the symptoms disappear."

GALL BLADDER FUNCTION ENERGY

> Body of objective thought;
>
> controls man's personal
>
> decisions and mental
>
> reactions.

Shortly after emerging at the center of the lower eyelid, the Gall Bladder Function Energy divides itself into two parts, A and B. (See Figure 6.21.)

Part A circulates the cheekbone before ascending to a point a quarter-inch from the outer edge of the eyebrow. At that point, the energy describes a half-circle around the back of the ear toward the earlobe. Part A then turns toward the back of the head and ascends in another half-circle to the forehead. Upon reaching the forehead, the flow travels in yet another semicircle toward the back of the head, where it splits into two parts, 1 and 2.

Part 1 flows to the acromion (the front of shoulder-and-arm joint). Part 2 flows from the first thoracic vertebra (at the top of the back), diagonally to the rear of the shoulder joint. From the joint, 2 descends to the hollow of the acromion. It then continues into the chest, where it crosses Gall Bladder Function Energy part B before descending to the seventh front rib cartilage. At the seventh rib, 2 intermingles briefly with B again be-

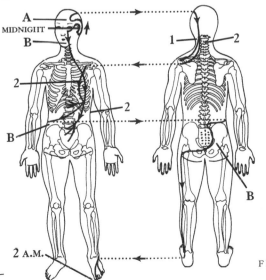

FIGURE 6.21

fore splitting into two branches. One of these branches of 2 flows to the stomach; the other flows to the umbilicus and scatters.

Part B, meanwhile, has descended from the cheekbone to the front of the shoulder, through the front of the fourth rib, and on to the seventh rib cartilage, where it comes to intermingle with part 2 of the A flow.

Remember that there are two sets of all the various branches of the gall bladder flow mirroring each other down the left and right sides of the body. However, along part B, the left and right pathways flow through different organs. The left part B travels through the liver, the gall bladder, and then on to the fourth lumbar. The right part B goes through the spleen and pancreas en route to the fourth lumbar. From the fourth lumbar, the left and right parts B continue on into the abdomen. Leaving the abdomen, both flows circulate around the pelvis and then emerge at the opposite side of the rectum. Continuing along the opposite side buttocks, each flow descends along the outer side of the legs and into the outer ankle, where it separates into two parts. One part flows across the top of the foot to the ring toe. The other part flows diagonally across the top of the foot to the big toenail, where it becomes the Liver Function Energy.

The Gall Bladder Function Energy is at its peak between the hours of midnight and two A.M. and during the spring season.

Anger is the attitude associated with disharmony of the gall bladder flow.

To Balance the Gall Bladder Flow

The third depth creates the gall bladder flow. The gall bladder flow is therefore harmonized by jumper-cabling the middle finger.

The following exercise can also be used:

1. Place your left hand on the left SEL 12 (at the back of the neck, midway between the skull and the shoulders). At the

same time, use your
right hand to jumper-
cable the right SEL
20 (on the upper
forehead, slightly
above the eyebrows).
(See Figure 6.22.)

2. Place your right hand
on the right SEL 12
(at the back of the
neck, midway
between the skull and
the shoulders). At the
same time, use your
left hand to jumper-
cable the left SEL 20 (on the upper forehead, slightly above
the eyebrows).

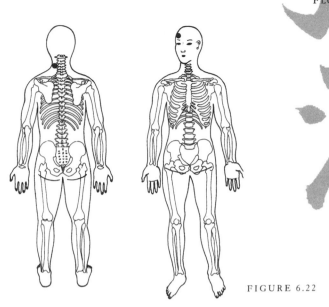

FIGURE 6.22

*"A SCHOOLTEACHER FROM Los Angeles was scheduled to go
to Europe the next day, but she had a terrible migraine
headache and didn't think she'd be able to go. She was
talking to her friend on the phone about it, and he said, 'You
need a Jin Shin Jyutsu session,' and gave her my number.
She called, and I said, 'I'll meet you at my office.' She was in
too much pain to drive, so her mother brought her in. She
was really having a rough time.*

*"I REMEMBERED HOW Mary said the gall bladder flow was
very good for clearing out migraines, so that's what I used. At
the end of that flow, she said, 'The pain is almost gone!
Nothing like this has ever happened before!' And at the end of
the session she was peaceful and ecstatic. 'I can't believe this,'
she said. 'Now I can go to Europe.' When she came back, she
began to study Jin Shin Jyutsu, and now she's a practitioner."*

LIVER FUNCTION ENERGY

Binds the soul to the body.

At two A.M., from the inner side of the big toenail, the Liver Func-tion Energy ascends through the inner ankle, up the leg through the groin, and into the pubic area. (See Figure 6.23.) The left flow ascends through the right side of the abdomen and the right side of the stomach before entering the gall bladder. The right flow as-cends the left side of the abdomen and the stomach on its way into the pancreas.

Both the right and left flows then move through the diaphragm and separate into three parts, A, B, and C. Part A ascends and then crosses over to the first front rib and the underarm area, then scat-ters and flows into the pleura. Part B crosses over to the opposite side of the throat, where it moves up to the back of the eye. After moving up through the cerebrum, it turns down along the back of the head and into the esophagus, then scatters at the outer side of the stomach.

Part C flows into the lungs and becomes the Lung Function En-ergy, thus completing the cycle that began twenty-four hours ago.

The Liver Function Energy is at its peak between the hours of two and four A.M. and during the spring season.

The attitude associated with disharmony of the liver flow en-ergy is anger.

To Balance the Liver Flow

By holding one of the middle fingers, you can balance the third depth, which in turn balances the liver flow. Or you can directly re-vitalize the flow itself with this simple "quickie":

1. Hold the left SEL 4 (at the base of the skull) with your left hand, while holding the right SEL 22 (under the

collarbone) with your right hand. (See Figure 6.24.)

2. Hold the right SEL 4 (at the base of the skull) with your right hand, while holding the left SEL 22 (under the collarbone) with your left hand.

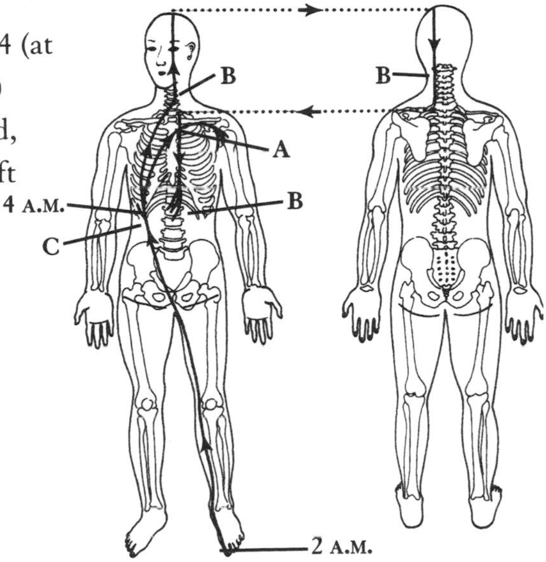

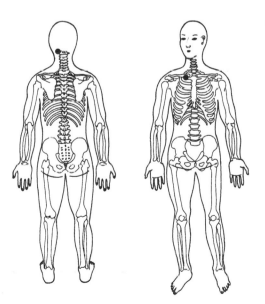

FIGURE 6.23

"ONE DAY WHILE working as a home health care nurse, I was seeing my own patients and covering for another nurse who was on vacation. I was sent to a man named Timothy, who was dying of liver cancer. Timothy, an elderly Irish gentleman, was lying on his couch looking pale and emaciated, in severe pain, with a massively distended abdomen and short of breath at rest. Timothy indicated to me that his greatest concern was that his daughter was being married on Saturday (three or four days away), and he was afraid he would not

FIGURE 6.24

be able to walk her down the aisle, since he could not even walk the several feet from his couch to the door. I asked if he was interested in experiencing an energy harmonizing art I knew to see what happened. He agreed. Each day for three or four days, I quickly performed my conventional nursing duties and went to work on energy harmonizing. I used the Liver Function Energy. Timothy's energy improved daily, and his symptoms were partially relieved. The wedding was the next day. I said good-bye and wished him well.

"I RECEIVED A call the following Tuesday from his wife. She said that her husband had not only walked his daughter down the aisle but had danced with her at the reception. He died a couple of days later. Before he died, Timothy said to his wife, 'Tell Pattie, it was because of her and the Jin Shin Jyutsu. Tell her thank you.' Of course, I was amazed and deeply thankful for him and his family. For myself, I not only got to be involved in this man's journey, I believe this experience was the reason I remained in home health care."

Collectively, the twelve organ flows constitute an amazingly comprehensive network that conveys nourishing energy to every region of our body, twenty-four hours a day. As we continue to heighten our awareness of the energy routes that make up this network, we can better understand that we are not just a collection of interlocking parts but a glorious, unified whole. Moreover, the better we comprehend the manifold relationships that exist between the various flows, the safety energy locks, and the depths, the more "immunized" we are against the fear of the unknown—a fear we might ordinarily feel when confronted with "big scary labels." It enables us to realize that a big lung project, for example, does not necessarily indicate an irreparably damaged lung. Rather, we learn to perceive it as a large but correctable disruption of energy somewhere along the network that nourishes the lungs.

Of course, if we faithfully practice the finger holds and "quickie" exercises presented throughout this chapter, we may never reach the point of dealing with many of those "big scary labels." We were already well acquainted with how the finger holds help us maintain an overall sense of well-being by balancing the all-encompassing depths. Now we also have at our disposal twelve "quickies" that allow us to directly jumper-cable SELs located along a particular organ flow. Using these SELs enables us to jumper-cable any energy that might be stuck at some point along that flow. (It should be noted that these "quickies" are shortened versions of longer Jin Shin Jyutsu exercises for balancing each of the twelve flows. These exercises, which often involve jumper-cabling a number of different SELs along the flow, can be rather detailed and are thus beyond the range of this book. Anyone interested in learning more about them is encouraged to attend an authorized Jin Shin Jyutsu class.)

In the next chapter we will present three very special and powerful exercises that can specifically help to revitalize our spleen, stomach and bladder flows. Yet they are also excellent for maintaining a overall sense of well-being and for providing a quick boost of energy. As such, they are recommended for everyday use and are often referred to as the general daily sequences.

general daily sequences

The daily sequences are complete because they clean the total front and the total back.

The twelve organ flows, along with the depths, the Trinity Flows, and the safety energy locks, are the concepts that form the core of the Jin Shin Jyutsu healing art. After an initial exposure to these concepts, it is not uncommon for students to be astonished at the seemingly endless number of ways in which their subtle interactions can influence almost any aspect of the body, mind, and spirit. But

133

upon first encountering these concepts, many people find themselves feeling somewhat overwhelmed. Often new levels of awareness will induce a sense of confusion if we attempt to comprehend unfamiliar ideas using old, familiar formulas. In her classes, Mary has often reminded new students that "confusion is progress."

Along similar lines, many of us who lead busy lives may have also wondered about the practicality of learning and integrating all of these new concepts and practices into an already-full schedule. The general daily sequences described in this chapter serve as a practical and effective solution to this particular dilemma. Not only are they easy to learn, but they are quite helpful in unloading much of the "dirt, dust and greasy grime" that can accumulate during the course of a busy lifestyle. For this reason, they are often referred to as the "janitors."

Each one of these three janitors serves to clean up a different range of energy within the body. These ranges are referred to as the Anterior Ascending Energy, the Anterior Descending Energy, and the Posterior Descending Energy. Revitalizing all three in succession is an especially good way to deal with almost all of the various stresses that we regularly confront in modern life. Moreover, all three of these sequences may be just as easily applied to oneself as to another, which makes them particularly good for self-help purposes. For all of these reasons, they are particularly recommended for everyday use.

In applying the sequences, just follow the same procedure that you have followed up until now. Simply hold each position for a few minutes, or until a pulsation or a deep sense of overall relaxation is felt. At that point, move on to the next step. It may be difficult to feel the rhythm of the pulse change at first, but with practice you will find yourself growing increasingly sensitive to it.

If time permits, use the sequences for both the left and right sides of the body, or simply jumper-cable the side of the body where there is more tension. There are no rigid rules. It is okay to adjust a sequence to whatever feels most convenient and comfortable. If, for instance, a particular step feels especially revitalizing, use that step regularly. It can serve as a personalized "quickie" revitalizing exercise. Finally, remember that there is an effective three-inch radius surrounding each area. You need not be overly concerned with precision. The body's wisdom knows how to use the energy channeled through the depths, flows, and safety energy locks. A close approximation to the location described in the sequence is sufficient to send an abundant flow of life energy through the appropriate safety energy lock.

ANTERIOR ASCENDING ENERGY SEQUENCE

This particular sequence works to revitalize the Spleen Function Energy. In Jin Shin Jyutsu the spleen is often regarded as a source of the body's "solar energy." As such, this sequence will deliver an excellent energy boost when you feel run down or fatigued. Since the spleen flow, when harmonized, also serves to alleviate worry, this sequence is quite good for calming the nerves. It also serves to strengthen the digestive function.

For the *right* side of the body (see Figure 7.1):

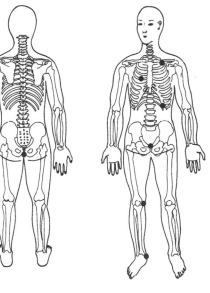

1. Place your left hand (the palm side or the back of the hand, whichever is most comfortable) at the base of the spine (coccyx).

2. Place your right hand on the *right* SEL 5,

FIGURE 7.1

between the inside ankle bone and the inside heel. (See diagram.) (If this position is uncomfortable, place the right fingers on the *right* inside of the knee or on the pubic bone.)

3. Move your right hand to the *left* SEL 14, at the base of the *left* front rib cage, at the center.

4. Move your left hand to the *right* SEL 13, at the center of the *right* third rib down from the collarbone (clavicle), just above the right breast area.

5. Move your left hand to the *left* SEL 22, at the center of the *left* collarbone.

For the *left* side of the body (see Figure 7.2):
The sequence is the reverse of the sequence for the right.

1. Place your right hand (the palm side or the back of the hand, whichever is most comfortable) at the base of the spine (coccyx).

2. Place your left hand on the *left* SEL 5, between the inside ankle bone and the heel. (See diagram.) (If this position is uncomfortable, place the left fingers on the *left* inside of the knee or on the pubic bone.)

3. Move your left hand to the *right* SEL 14, at the base of the *right* front rib cage. (The right hand is still at the base of the spine.)

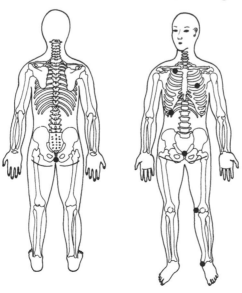

FIGURE 7.2

4. Move your right hand to the *left* SEL 13, at the center of the *left* third rib, below the left collarbone (clavicle), right above the left breast area.

5. Move your right hand to the *right* SEL 22, at the center of the *right* collarbone.

> "*I HAVE ALWAYS had a sweet tooth. As a result, I periodically find myself eating way more sugar than is good for me. Afterward, I often wind up feeling either too jittery or very sluggish.*
>
> "*A FEW YEARS ago, at a friend's recommendation, I attended a Jin Shin Jyutsu self-help class, where I learned about the Anterior Ascending Energy sequence. I found myself recalling this sequence shortly after a subsequent sugar binge. I promptly began to apply it to myself. In a short while, I felt myself calmer and less fatigued. Since then, I have used this sequence daily. Not only do I feel an overall increase in energy, but my craving for sweets also seems to have diminished.*"

ANTERIOR DESCENDING ENERGY SEQUENCE

The following sequence will revitalize the energy that descends along the front of the body from head to toe. It works directly upon the Stomach Function Energy. Thus, like the previous sequence, it helps to relieve worry and mental stress. It is also quite effective for clearing any congestion that occurs above the waist, such as bloat. Accordingly, it is useful for assisting anyone involved with a weight project.

Remember   any step that you cannot reach comfortably can be skipped. Simply go on to the next step that you can apply without straining.

For the *right* side of the body (see Figure 7.3):

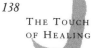

1. Place your left finger or fingers at the *right* SEL 21, at the base of the *right* cheekbone. Keep it there for the remainder of the sequence.

2. Place your right finger or fingers at the center of the *right* SEL 22, at the collarbone.

3. Move your right finger or fingers to the *left* SEL 14, at the base of the center of the *left* front rib cage.

4. Move your right finger or fingers to the *left* SEL 23, at the small of the back.

5. Move your right finger or fingers to the *right* SEL 14, at the base of the center of the *right* front rib cage.

6. Move your right finger or fingers to the *left* high SEL 1, on the inside of the *left* thigh, about three inches above the left knee.

7. Move your right finger or fingers halfway down the left calf—to the low SEL 8, about midway between the outside of the knee and ankle—off the *left* shinbone.

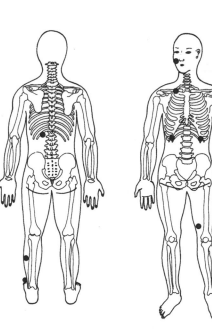

8. Move your right finger or fingers to the *left* middle toe and hold the middle toe with the finger and thumb.

FIGURE 7.3

Note: Your left finger or fingers have been on the base of the right cheekbone throughout this sequence, and only your right finger or fingers have moved.

For the *left* side of the body (see Figure 7.4):

The sequence is the reverse of the sequence for the right side. As time permits, both the right and left sequences may be applied. However, if time does not permit, jumper-cable only the side that has more tension.

1. Place your right finger or fingers on the *left* SEL 21, at the base of the *left* cheekbone.

2. Place your left finger or fingers at the *left* SEL 22, at the center of the *left* collarbone.

3. Move your left finger or fingers to the *right* SEL 14, at the base of the center of the *right* front rib cage.

4. Move your left finger or fingers to the *right* SEL 23, at the small of the back.

5. Move your left finger or fingers to the *left* SEL 14, at the base of the center of the *left* front rib cage.

6. Move your left finger or fingers to the *right* high SEL 1, on the inside of the *right* thigh, about three inches above the right knee.

7. Move your left finger or fingers halfway

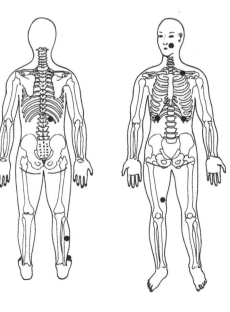

FIGURE 7.4

down to the right calf—to the low SEL 8, midway
between the outside of the knee and off the *right* shinbone.

8. Move your left finger or fingers to the *right* middle toe.
Hold the middle toe with the finger and thumb.

> "BEFORE I WAS introduced to Jin Shin Jyutsu, I had little or
> no control over my periodic bouts with indigestion, which
> were caused by my allergies to certain foods and preservatives.
> Although I had tried various prescription medications for
> dealing with the problem, they all had side effects that I found
> undesirable.
>
> "IN 1979 A good friend of mine was with me when I was
> suffering from one of these attacks. I felt as if a tight band had
> been wound around my chest, hampering my breathing. From
> past experience, I knew my symptoms were stomach related
> and that I would be in for several hours of severe discomfort
> and nausea.
>
> "FORTUNATELY, MY FRIEND was a Jin Shin Jyutsu
> practitioner. She immediately began to work on me. Imagine
> my surprise and delight when all of my symptoms disappeared
> within thirty minutes! I couldn't believe it would last. I asked
> my friend if these same results could be consistently repeated.
> She told me that they could and that I even had the ability to
> do it myself.
>
> "SHE PROCEEDED TO show me something called the Anterior
> Descending Energy Sequence that I could use to help my
> stomach. For the past fifteen years, I have used this sequence
> daily. It has come to my rescue on many occasions."

POSTERIOR DESCENDING ENERGY SEQUENCE

This sequence acts upon the Bladder Function Energy. Therefore, it is useful for facilitating the body's elimination processes. It is also a powerful tool for clearing up headaches and back stress, as well as muscle and leg discomforts.

For the *right* side of the body (see Figure 7.5):

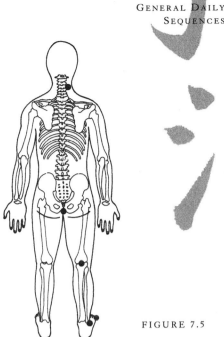

FIGURE 7.5

1. Place your left finger or fingers on the *right* SEL 12, at the side of the neck between the ear and spine.

2. Place your right hand (the back of the hand or the palm side) on the base of the spine, at the coccyx.

3. Move your right finger or fingers to the back of the *right* knee, at the center (where the knee bends).

4. Move your right finger or fingers to the *right* SEL 16, on the right outside of the ankle, below the *right* ankle bone.

5. Move your right finger or fingers to the *right* little toe, and hold the little toe with the thumb and finger.

For the *left* side of the body (see Figure 7.6): The sequence is the reverse of the sequence for the *right*.

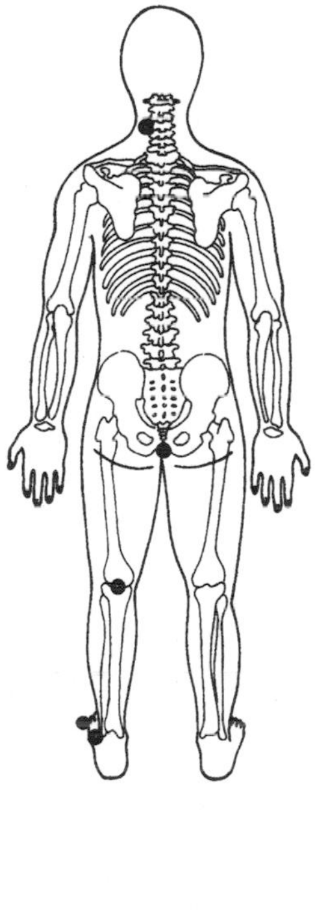

FIGURE 7.6

1. Place your right finger or fingers on the *left* SEL 12, at the left side of the neck, between the ear and the spine.

2. Place your left hand (the back of the hand or the palm) on the base of the spine, at the coccyx.

3. Move your left finger or fingers to the back of the *left* knee, at the center (where the knee bends).

4. Move your left finger or fingers to the *left* SEL 16, on the left outside of the ankle, below the *left* ankle bone.

5. Move your left finger or fingers to the *left* little toe, and hold the little toe with the thumb and finger.

"I'D EXPERIENCED SCIATIC pain all the way down my right leg. This pain continued nonstop for nearly two years, ever since my seventh month of pregnancy. The discomfort was always present—sometimes a searing pain that kept me up at night, at other times a dull ache.

"AFTER RECEIVING MY first Jin Shin Jyutsu treatment, the practitioner sent me home with instructions to use the self-help bladder flow twice daily [that is, the Posterior Descending Energy Sequence]. I followed her directions, going through the flow for about fifteen minutes each morning and evening. At the end of five days, there was no more discomfort at all. I also felt distinctly calmer and more optimistic.

"FOR THE NEXT six or seven years, I never experienced even a hint of pain. In the past few years, on several occasions, a slight ghost of the ache has reminded me of the pathway of the sciatic nerve. One or two applications of the self-help bladder flow always clears it right up."

The preceding sequences are among the most powerful self-help tools in the entire Jin Shin Jyutsu repertoire. For those whose lifestyles may be especially hectic, these three general daily sequences cannot be recommended highly enough. However, anyone who chooses to make them a part of their everyday routine will gain immediate and lasting benefits. Simply by allowing ourselves a few minutes daily for their application, we revitalize and nourish those parts of ourselves that consistently endure the greatest stress.

harmonizing with the fingers and toes

As we saw back in Chapter 1, when Jiro Murai was pronounced incurably ill, he retreated to his family's mountain cabin. There he fasted, meditated, and performed various finger postures, which are known as mudras. *Murai's experience with these mudras led him toward the insights that resulted in Jin Shin Jyutsu. In a sense, then, everything*

It is comforting to know that all the things we need to be in harmony with the universe—our fingers and toes—are with us at all times. We need never fear that we have forgotten or misplaced them.

that we have learned in the preceding seven chapters can be traced back to those simple finger postures. When we take the time to learn and practice these mudras, we not only reacquaint ourselves with the roots of the art, we also acquire powerful tools for the restoration of health and tranquillity.

Earlier, too, we noted that each of our ten fingers can regulate 14,400 functions within the body. Murai learned that bending, stretching, and clasping the ten fingers in various ways can create as many as 680 different mudras. It is not hard to imagine, then, that a knowledge of these various mudras could allow us to send energy to any part of our being. Murai also believed that the simple act of joining the left and right hands could bring about a unity between the body and mind. Ultimately, therefore, the mudras can give us the ability to address a wide array of mental and emotional issues, including those that manifest themselves as a concern for our physical condition.

Immediately following are eight particularly powerful mudras that empower us to address both the causes and concerns relevant to a number of different disharmonies.

FINGER POSE 1: EXHALING THE BURDENS AND BLOCKAGES

Hold the palm side of the left middle finger lightly with the right thumb. Place the rest of the right-hand fingers on the back side of the left middle finger. (See Figure 8.1.) Reverse for the right middle finger, in the same way.

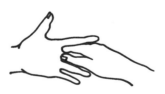

This finger pose aids in releasing generalized tension and stress from head to toe. It facilitates our exhalation, which in turn

FIGURE 8.1

allows us to empty ourselves of the causes of harmful stagnation and blockages of energy.

In addition, this mudra can be used whenever you find yourself beset with any of these particular concerns:

- I can't see too well.

- I have a hard time exhaling.

- I get frustrated.

- I'm tired all the time.

- I have trouble making up my mind—I'm a procrastinator.

FINGER POSE 2: INHALING THE ABUNDANCE

Hold the back of the left middle finger lightly with the right thumb. Place the other fingers of the right hand on the palm side of the left middle finger. (See Figure 8.2.) Reverse this procedure for the right middle finger.

This finger pose promotes easier inhaling of the Breath of Life—our source of abundance. It can be used to alleviate the following mental or physical concerns:

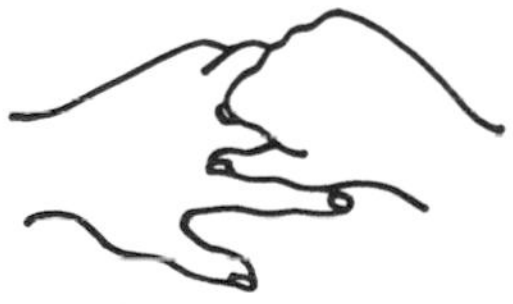

FIGURE 8.2

- I can't "take" a deep breath.

- I'm getting hard of hearing.

- My feet are bothering me.

- I'm not as alert as I used to be.

- My eyes are really bothering me.

FINGER POSE 3: CALMING AND REVITALIZING

Hold the palm side of the left little and ring fingers with the right thumb. Place the other right fingers on the back of the left little and ring fingers. (See Figure 8.3.) Reverse for the right fingers.

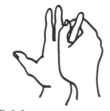

FIGURE 8.3

This finger pose aids in calming the body, releasing nervous tension and stress, and revitalizing all of the organ functions. It can be used whenever you feel any of the following states of mind or physical symptoms:

- I get so nervous.

- I worry about my heart.

- I can't walk too much without getting out of breath.

- I'm always "trying-to."

- I get so depressed, I have no *fun*.

FINGER POSE 4: RELEASING GENERAL DAILY FATIGUE

Hold the back of the left thumb, index, and middle fingers with the right thumb. Place the rest of the right fingers on the palm side of the left thumb, index, and middle fingers. (See Figure 8.4.) Reverse for the right thumb and fingers.

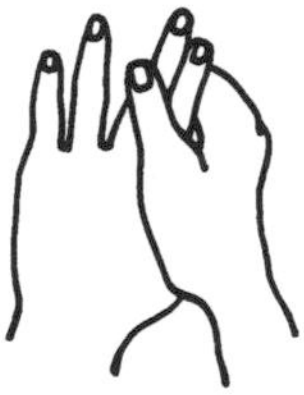

FIGURE 8.4

This finger pose aids in releasing the fatigue, tension, and stress that can build up during the course of daily life. It assists in the release of worries, fears, and anger. It

can be used to ease any of the following mental or physical difficulties:

- I get so tired.

- I feel insecure about everything—my health, my wealth, my happiness.

- I'm beginning to feel old and look old.

- I get irritated and angry over nothing.

- I worry about everything.

Finger Pose 5: Total Revitalization

Make a circle with the right middle finger and thumb by placing the palm side of the thumb on the middle fingernail. Next, slip the left thumb between the circle of the right thumb and middle finger. (See Figure 8.5.) Reverse for the right side.

This mudra aids in the revitalization of all bodily functions and releases those blockages that are responsible for daily fatigue. It also assists in overcoming any of the following conditions:

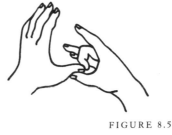

FIGURE 8.5

- I always have an uneasy feeling.

- Nothing seems to be wrong with me, but I get tired all the time.

- My complexion is terrible.

- I'm temperamental—I just can't help it.

- I have an uncontrollable craving for sweets.

FINGER POSE 6: BREATHING FREELY

Touch the right ring fingernail with the palm side of the thumb and hold for several minutes. (See Figure 8.6.) Reverse for left ring finger and thumb.

This finger pose strengthens the respiratory function and helps to balance all ear-related projects. When used while walking, jogging, running, or exercising, this finger pose helps us to breathe more easily. It also can be utilized when flying or driving in high altitudes. Use this finger pose whenever any of the following physical or emotional conditions are predominant:

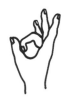

FIGURE 8.6

- My skin condition is terrible.

- I feel rejected and unloved and get teary easily.

- I'm all thumbs. I'm just plain clumsy.

- I've lost all of my common sense.

- My ears are bothering me.

Finger Poses 7 and 8 help us bring harmony to the total being.

FINGER POSE 7: EXHALING THE DIRT, DUST, AND GREASY GRIME

Touch the palm sides of the left and right middle fingers in the folded hands position. (See Figure 8.7.)

This finger pose aids in releasing general daily tension and stress

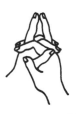

FIGURE 8.7

from the head, lungs, digestive functions, abdomen, and legs. It also strengthens the ability to exhale and unloads any accumulated dirt, dust, and greasy grime.

FINGER POSE 8: INHALING THE PURIFIED BREATH OF LIFE

Bring the left and right middle fingernails together. (See Figure 8.8.)

This finger pose helps to release the tension in the back and promotes an overall feeling of well-being. It also strengthens our ability to inhale and receive the purified breath of life.

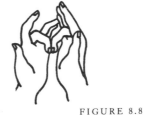

FIGURE 8.8

Besides these mudras, the hands can also be used in conjunction with the feet to address a wide array of disharmonies affecting body, mind, and spirit. These hand and feet sequences are explored below.

the link between
the hands and feet

On the most obvious levels, the hands and feet bear striking similarities in shape, from the heel of the hand to heel of the foot; from the thumb to the big toe. Traditional healers see these similarities as the result of corresponding energy patterns. As a result, they have long seen the hands and feet as being energetically linked.

After years of experimentation and research, Jiro Murai observed that the top-third segments of the fingers and toes correspond to the upper part of the body—the mental and emotional functions, the brain, and the chest. He noted that this same set of joints corresponds to the thighs. When the upper joints of the fingers and toes are jumper-cabled, any mental or emotional stresses, as well as tension in the chest and thighs, can be relieved.

The middle joints in both fingers and toes correspond to the face, digestive functions, abdomen, and calves. Jumper-cabling these middle joints helps relieve any blockages in these areas. Finally, the bottom joints of the fingers and toes correspond to the neck, pelvis, and feet, as well as to the overall physical body. When we jumper-cable the bottom joints, energy is directed to these areas.

Jiro Murai also saw a similar relationship between the three sets of digit joints and the palms of the hands and the soles of the feet. The upper-third joints correspond to the upper palms and soles. Similarly, the middle joints of the digits correspond to the center of the palms and soles. The lower joints of the fingers and toes conform to the heels of the hands and feet.

Jin Shin Jyutsu also recognizes that there is an analogous relationship between the opposite fingers and toes. These relationships will become more apparent if you place one hand over the opposite foot. This way you can see how the thumb lines up with the little toe, the index finger with the ring toe, and so on.

What follows are self-help sequences that utilize these relationships between the hands and feet to help restore health and harmony.

THE PALMS AND SOLES: REVITALIZING THE ENTIRE BEING

The centers of the palms and the soles are related to the Main Central Flow, the source of our life energy. This energy, which

nourishes all the cells of the body, can therefore be harmonized using the palms and soles. Often people clench their hands unconsciously to help themselves regenerate and revitalize their fatigued and run-down condition. Clenched hands signify much tension and stress, whereas open palms suggest a more relaxed state of being.

The following two sequences can be used to alleviate exhaustion, mental confusion, eye strain, and abdominal cramping. They also help circulation in the feet.

The Palms

Place the palm sides of your hands together, so that your right fingertips touch the left palm and your left fingertips touch the right palm. (See Figure 8.9.)

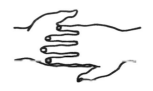

FIGURE 8.9

The Soles of the Feet

With your left hand, hold the left foot in such a way that your fingertips touch the center of the sole, while your thumb holds the top of the foot. (See Figure 8.10.) You can jumper-cable one foot at a time or both feet simultaneously.

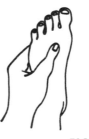

FIGURE 8.10

OPPOSITE FINGERS AND TOES

The Thumbs and the Little Toes

The "needy" thumbs and little toes are often the most sensitive digits to jumper-cable. Accordingly, they frequently need the most recharging and the most loving care.

Jin Shin Jyutsu regards the thumbs as the "leaders of the parade." If the thumb energy is not in rhythm, then all that follows will be out of step.

The thumbs dissipate general daily fatigue and promote healthy digestive function. By jumper-cabling either one, we can release tension from the head, shoulders, and lungs.

The little toes harmonize all forms of muscle cramping and help to eliminate headaches. They release fear, insecurity, uncertainty, jealousy, feelings of revenge, and stubbornness.

By jumper-cabling the little toes, you can release tension from the back and promote healthy assimilation and elimination and stronger reproductive functions. (See Figure 8.11.) The little toes also strengthen the kidney and bladder functions.

Like the mudras, these finger and toe sequences can be used to alleviate mental stresses regarding physical conditions. The thumb-and-little-toe sequence can be used whenever you find yourself thinking any of the following:

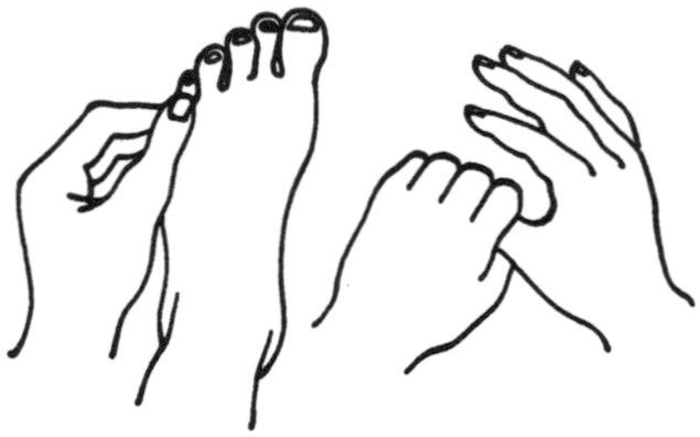

FIGURE 8.11

- I'm out of balance.

- I have a hard time breathing.

- My heartbeat is irregular.

- I have a fever.

- My digestive system is out of balance.

- I feel nervous.

- I have muscle spasms.

- I tire easily.

- I'm a worrier.

- I'm insecure and unsure of myself.

- I can't seem to lose weight.

- I feel bloated.

The Index Fingers and Ring Toes

By jumper-cabling the index fingers, you can affect the functions that revitalize the bones and bone marrow. (See Figure 8.12.) Jumper-cabling the index fingers helps babies eliminate discomforts related to teething and drooling; promotes healing of teeth and gums; prevents graying and thinning of hair; and promotes healthy circulation throughout the body.

Holding the index fingers and ring toes help to reduce fear and depression. It is also useful for the release of blockages that cause bloating, fluid retention, and gas.

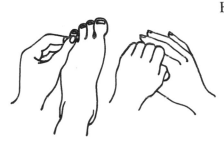

FIGURE 8.12

The ring toes by themselves can be jumper-cabled to revitalize the liver, gall bladder, spleen, pancreas, and diaphragm functions. Also, the back and the respiratory system can be strengthened through their application.

Hold the ring toes and the index fingers whenever you find yourself thinking:

- I'm insecure and afraid.

- I feel negative.

- I feel lonely and unloved.

- I can't seem to get ahead. I'm always in need.

- I'm bored.

- I'm constipated.

- I have chronic ear problems.

- I have bursitis, tennis elbow, and wrist and/or finger pains.

- My nails look terrible.

The Middle Toes and the Middle Fingers

Jumper-cabling the middle toes and the middle fingers is a general harmonizer, but it is especially powerful for the respiratory and digestive functions. (See Figure 8.13.) It promotes optimal and healthy production of milk for mothers who are breastfeeding. It releases tension and stress from the knees.

This exercise is useful when you are experiencing any of the following:

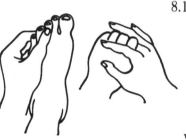

FIGURE 8.13

- I'm angry.

- I'm tired. I look haggard.

- I bruise easily.

- I have migraines.

- My eyes are giving me problems.

- I can't breathe.

- My digestion is giving me problems.

- I have swallowing problems.

- I have speech problems.

- I have hearing problems.

- I'm always hyper—I can't relax.

The Index Toes and the Ring Fingers

By holding the index toes and the ring fingers, we can release tension and stress in the chest, breathing, and digestive system. (See Figure 8.14.) This is also excellent for restoring joy to one's being, clearing the mind, and improving eyesight.

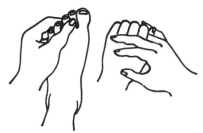

Use this sequence whenever you feel:

FIGURE 8.14

- I'm out of harmony.

- My emotions are shot.

- I'm unhappy and can't seem to get myself out of it.

- I'm a victim of my thoughts, my feelings, my desires. I can't even breathe, my chest is so tight. I'm full of mucus.

- I sound weepy even when I'm not sad.

- I'm just a sorry mess. I have skin problems, rashes, and excess body hair.

- My eyes are bothering me.

- I have digestive problems.

- I have no energy, but the more I lie around, the worse I feel.

The Big Toes and Little Fingers

The little fingers and big toes harmonize the circulatory, nervous, muscular, and skeletal systems. They also aid in relieving ear

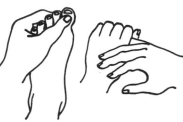

FIGURE 8.15

problems and digestive stress. (See Figure 8.15.) Jumper-cabling the little fingers and big toes can bring laughter into our lives. It can also reduce bloating or ankle swelling. If you find yourself unable to think clearly or if you suffer from headaches or respiratory problems, holding the little fingers and big toes can provide the remedy.

Also hold these fingers and toes whenever you feel:

- I'm so embarrassed when I start stuttering. I panic, and that doesn't help matters.

- I perspire so, it's embarrassing.

- I'm thirsty all the time.

- I try so hard, but I can't seem to make much headway, and I get discouraged.

- How can I be happy, anyway?

- I'm getting varicose veins, and they're beginning to hurt and look ugly.

- I have digestive problems and heartburn, which worry me.

- My hearing is getting bad.

- I have a ringing in my ears.

- My skin is dry.

- I don't seem to have any enthusiasm or joy.

- I guess I'll never succeed. I am a failure.

- I try walking to build up my strength, but I feel worse after my walks.

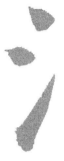

- My baby has trouble sleeping.

- I broke my leg.

- I sprained my ankle.

- I'm accident-prone.

- I have urinary problems.

- I have no energy.

- I have a sweet tooth.

The creative power of the entire universe lies within each one of these fingers and toes. The only way we can know this, however, is to experience the transformation that takes place when we actually jumper-cable them. We can be our own testimony and see for ourselves what beautiful and dynamic tools we are endowed with.

first aid and on-the-spot healing

chapter nine

*T*hroughout this book, we have seen a

wide range of applications for Jin Shin

Jyutsu. It can be used as a preventive

measure, and it can be used to relieve

chronic, longstanding conditions. Jin

Shin Jyutsu is also quite effective as first

aid in emergencies. Its immediate

accessibility allows us to use it for

situations requiring on-the-spot care. It

can be used when help is otherwise impossible to secure, such as during travel in remote areas. It is also beneficial as an adjunct to conventional methods of treatment. Its gentle, noninvasive nature assures that its application is safe and does not interfere with other treatments.

The following is a listing of the many ways in which Jin Shin Jyutsu can be applied either as first aid or for chronic conditions. These quickies may be used either for oneself or to assist others. Some of the sequences are repeated several times throughout the chapter—they are beneficial in a wide variety of situations.

Alertness—Sit on your hands, either on the palms or on the backs of the hands, while holding SEL 25, located at the ischium (sit-bones).

Allergies—Hold the high SEL 19 (at the upper arm) and the opposite SEL 1 (on the inner thigh).

Ankle and foot projects—Hold the wrist opposite the sore ankle at SEL 17.

Anxiety—Cross the arms and hold the outer edge of the shoulder blades, near the underarms, at SEL 26.

Appetite balance—Hold the base of the cheekbones at SEL 21.

Arthritis—While holding the left foot, hold SEL 5, at the inner ankle, with your right hand and SEL 16, at the outer ankle, with your left hand. For the right foot, hold SEL 5, at the inner ankle, with your right hand, and SEL 16, at the outer ankle, with your left hand. (See Figure 9.1.)

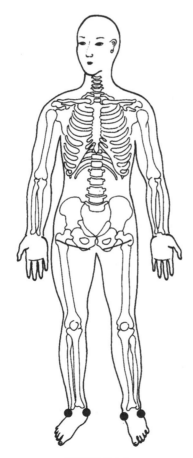

FIGURE 9.1

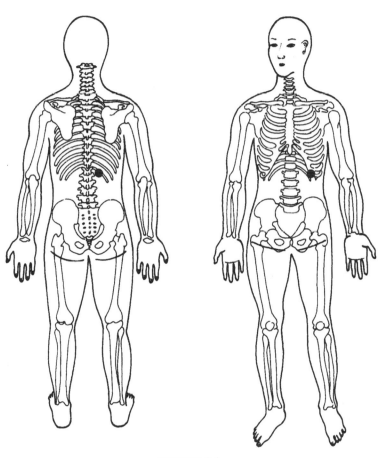

FIGURE 9.2

Asthma and breathing difficulties—With your left hand, hold the
base of the left rib cage at SEL 14, and with your right, hold the
right SEL 23, at the small of the back. (See Figure 9.2.)

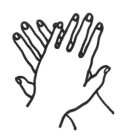

FIGURE 9.3

Backache and sciatica—Hold both the left and right SEL 15s, at the groin.

Bleeding—Place your right hand on the area of bleeding, and your left hand over the right hand. (See Figure 9.3.) Women who experience excessive menstrual flow can apply this hold to their lower abdominal area.

Bloating, swelling, and water retention—Cross your hands, and hold the inside of the knees at SEL 1.

Breast projects—Cross your arms, and hold the outer edge of the shoulder blades, near the underarms, at SEL 26.

Bunions—Hold the crease of the elbow at thumb-side SEL 19, and hold the same-side outer back of the knee at SEL 8. (See Figure 9.4.)

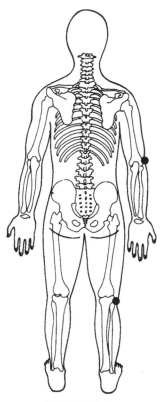

FIGURE 9.4

Burns—Palm the area, or
if that is too painful,
palm the area above the
burn (a few inches away
from the burned skin).
(See Figure 9.5.)

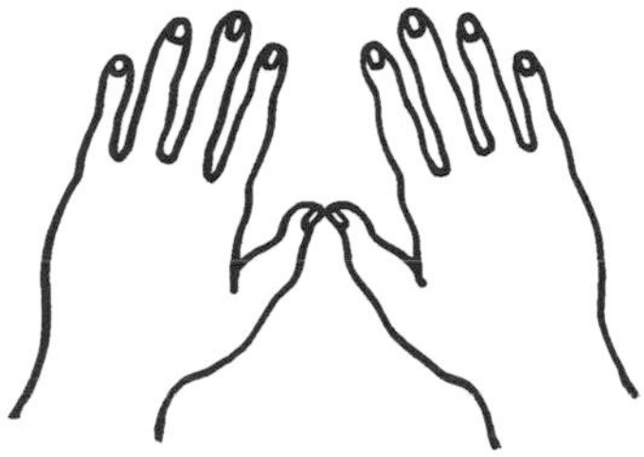

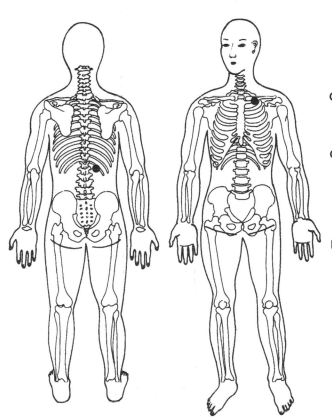

FIGURE 9.5

Cholesterol balance—Hold the center of the palm of your hands.

Chronic fatigue syndrome—Hold the small of the back on both
sides of the spine at SEL 23.

Colds, flu, and
fever—Hold the
upper shoulder, at
SEL 3, and the
same-side groin at
SEL 15.

Constipation—Hold
the left calf, at low
SEL 8.

Cramps and
spasms—Hold left
and right SEL 23,
at the small of the
back.

Depression—Hold
the area just
below the
collarbone, at SEL
22, and opposite
SEL 23, at the
small of the back.
(See Figure 9.6.)

FIGURE 9.6

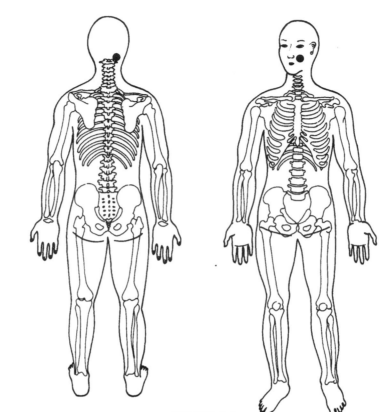

FIGURE 9.7

Diarrhea—Hold the right calf at low SEL 8.

Dizziness—Hold the base of the cheekbones at SEL 21.

Ear ringing—Hold the ring finger.

Eyestrain—Hold the back of the head, at SEL 4, and the opposite cheekbone, at SEL 21. (See Figure 9.7.)

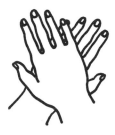

FIGURE 9.8

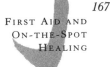

Fainting, unconsciousness—Hold the base of the skull at the SEL 4s.

Fertility—Hold both SEL 13s, at the chest.

Hammer toes—Palm the hammer toe, and hold the opposite arch at SEL 6.

Hangovers—Hold the upper shoulders and neck at SEL 11, SEL 12, and SEL 3.

Headaches:

Back-of-head headache—Hold the thumb at SEL 18.

Frontal headache—Hold the outer ankle at SEL 16.

Migraine—Hold both SEL 16 and SEL 18.

Hearing difficulties—Hold the shoulder at SEL 11, and the opposite chest at SEL 13.

Heartburn—Hold the area below the base of the sternum between the SEL 14s.

Heart conditions—Hold the little fingers.

Hiccups—Hold the area just behind the earlobes at lateral SEL 12.

Hot flashes—Hold the left calf at SEL 8.

Immune system—Hold the upper shoulder at SEL 3, and the same-side groin at SEL 15.

Impotency and sexual projects—Hold both sides at SEL 13, on the chest.

Insect bites—Place your left hand directly on the bite, and place your right hand over the left hand. (See Figure 9.8.) This hold can also be used for removing splinters.

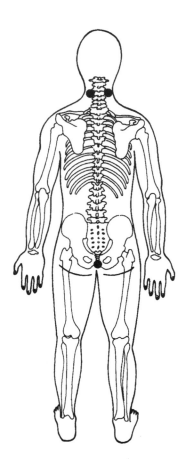

FIGURE 9.9

Insomnia—Hold the base of the thumb at SEL 18.

Jaw projects—Hold the painful jaw area and the opposite outer ankle at SEL 16.

Joint pain—Palm the area of joint discomfort.

Knee projects—Cross your arms, and hold your upper arms at high SEL 19.

Labor and delivery—Hold the lower back at SEL 2, and hold the opposite inside knee at SEL 1.

Memory—Place your right hand on top of the head, and place your left fingers between the eyebrows.

Menstrual tension—Hold both SELs 13 at the chest.

Muscle cramps—Hold the outer backs of the knees, at SEL 8.

Nausea—Cross your hands, and I hold high SEL 1 at the inner thighs.

Neck tension—Hold SEL 12 at the neck, and hold the base of the spine (coccyx). (See Figure 9.9.)

Nursing mothers—Hold the middle finger.

Reproductive projects (male and female)—Hold both sides of the chest, at SEL 13.

Shoulder tension—Hold the shoulder at SEL 11, and hold the same-side groin at SEL 15.

Sinus projects—Cross your arms, and hold SEL 19 by the crease of the elbow on the thumb side.

Skin projects (acne, rashes, etc.)—Palm both calves.

Tantrums—Hold the big toes, at SEL 7.

Toothache—Hold the index finger on the side opposite the painful tooth.

Wrist pain—Cross your arms, and hold SEL 19 by the crease of the elbow, on the thumb side.

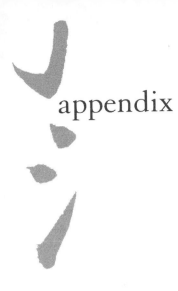

appendix

The following are the most frequently asked questions regarding the study and practice of Jin Shin Jyutsu.

How does one go about studying Jin Shin Jyutsu?

The Jin Shin Jyutsu basic five-day training is taught several times each year throughout the world. The seminar lasts thirty-five hours and combines combination lectures and hands-on training. Some students enroll intending to become practitioners, while others do so purely for personal reasons.

The training is comprised of two parts (*each with an accompanying text*):

In Part I (three days) the primary focus is on the vital relationship between invisible energy, how we breathe, the attitudes we hold, and their impact on the physical body. The concept of an invisible life energy is studied throughout the seminar. Continual reference is made to discerning the threefold nature of Man—spirit, mind, and body—and their interrelationships, and on understanding the role they play in our lives.

Besides a general introduction to Jin Shin Jyutsu, Part I describes its history and philosophy. It explains the Trinity

Flows and the Diagonal Mediators, the location of the twenty-six safety energy locks, and the sequences for harmonizing them and for balancing specific discordant energy patterns.

The main focus of Part II (two days) is on the manifested physical body. It introduces pulse listening and the twelve organ flows, including their circulation pathways, ways of restoring them to balance, and sequences for harmonizing specific imbalances.

How many Jin Shin Jyutsu instructors are there?

There are twelve instructors sanctioned by Mary Burmeister and by Jin Shin Jyutsu, Inc., to teach the five-day seminar and provide related materials.

Susan M. Brooks, Ph.D.

Muriel Carlton

Philomena Dooley

Carlos Gutterres

Wayne Hackett

Ian Kraut

Iole Lebensztajn

Brigitta Meinhardt

Lynne Pflueger

Waltraud Riegger-Krause

Mathias Roth

Jed Schwartz

In addition, Dr. Haruki Kato, a student of Master Jiro Murai, teaches Jin Shin Jyutsu to medical professionals in Japan.

Before the five-day seminar, is a basic foundational class of Jin Shin Jyutsu offered?

Many practitioners offer self-help Jin Shin Jyutsu classes that present the basic principles, based on Mary Burmeister's three introductory-level books.

Who teaches these classes?

Students who have completed three five-day seminars are qualified to attend the Instructor Training in Self-Help (IT IS) seminar. The IT IS seminar prepares interested students to conduct the self-help classes. A certificate of attendance is issued upon completion of the IT IS training. The instructors for the IT IS training are:

Sara Harper

Iole Lebensztajn

Brigitta Meinhardt

Janet Oliver

Phyllis Singer

Is it possible to get CEU credits by studying Jin Shin Jyutsu?

Continuing education credits are offered by EDUCARE, provider approved by the California Board of Registered Nursing, number 07359. Thirty contact hours are given for the basic seminar. Many other states recognize California CEUs.

Can one become a licensed Jin Shin Jyutsu practitioner?

No, Jin Shin Jyutsu, Inc., offers no formal license to practitioners. But a practitioner-level certificate is issued upon completion of three five-day seminars. At this point, the student has gained a basic understanding of Jin Shin Jyutsu and may embark upon a lifelong practice of the Art. As a general guideline, it is not recommended that students complete the three five-day seminars in less than eighteen months.

Where are Jin Shin Jyutsu seminars taught?

Currently, they are taught in almost half of the states in the United States, with the heaviest concentration of classes in the Arizona, California, Colorado, and New York areas. Jin Shin Jyutsu seminars are also offered in Brazil, Western Europe, and Canada.

For further information on seminars, materials, books, and lectures on Jin Shin Jyutsu in your area, please contact:

Jin Shin Jyutsu, Inc.

8719 East San Alberto

Scottsdale, Arizona 85258

tel. (480) 998-9331

fax: (480) 998-9335

website: www.jinshinjyutsu.com

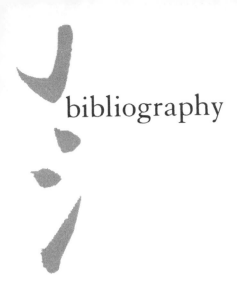

bibliography

Burmeister, Mary. *Introducing Jin Shin Jyutsu Is.* Books
1–3. Scottsdale, AZ: Jin Shin Jyutsu Distributors, 1981,
1985, 1994.

Burmeister, Mary. *Jin Shin Jyutsu Physio-Philosophy.* Texts
1 and 2. Scottsdale, AZ: Jin Shin Jyutsu, Inc., 1994.

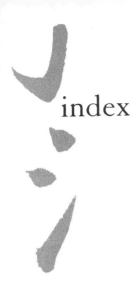

index

anger, 18
anterior ascending energy
    sequence, 134, 135–37
anterior descending energy
    sequence, 134, 137–40
attitudes, 18, 27
  anger, 18, 34
  fear, 18, 20, 36–37
  grief, 32, 33
  pretense, 18, 38–39
  total despondency, 28, 29
  worry, 18, 30
  See also depths

biorhythms, 100
Bladder Function Energy,
    115–17, 141
breath, 18, 19, 20–21, 40–41, 46

thirty-six breaths exercise,
  21
Burmeister, David, 7
Burmeister, Gil, 4, 15
Burmeister, Mary, 2, 4–5, 8, 9,
    11, 13, 16–17, 18, 20–21,
    23–24, 31, 37

conditions:
  first aid and on-the-spot
    healing, 161–69
  index of, with
    corresponding safety
    energy locks, 58
  See also attitudes; daily
    sequences; disharmonies
    (labels); finger poses
    (mudras); fingers and

toes; safety energy locks
(SELs)

daily sequences, 133–43
    anterior ascending energy,
        134, 135–37
    anterior descending energy,
        134, 137–40
    posterior descending energy,
        134, 141–42
depths, 18, 25–39, 100
    first, 27, 29–31, 57, 60–66
    second, 32–33, 57, 66–79
    third, 33–34, 57, 82–90
    fourth, 35–37, 57, 90–92
    fifth, 37–39, 57, 92–96
    sixth, 28–29, 45, 57
    seventh, 26
    eighth, 26
    ninth, 26
    safety energy locks and,
        56–57; *See also* safety
        energy locks (SELs)
    Supervisor Flows and, 49,
        56
    See also attitudes
Diagonal Mediator Flows,
    52
    project for harmonizing,
        52–54
Diaphragm Function Energy,
    120–22

disharmonies (labels), 18, 19,
    99–100, 130–31
    See also attitudes

eighth depth, 26
energy, life. *See* life energy

fear, 18, 20, 36–37
feet, hands linked with,
    151–59
    palms and soles: revitalizing
        the entire being, 152–53
    See also fingers and toes
fifth depth, 37–39, 57
    safety energy locks of, 92–
        96
finger poses (mudras), 145–51
    1 (exhaling the burdens and
        blockages), 146–47
    2 (inhaling the abundance),
        147
    3 (calming and revitalizing),
        148
    4 (releasing general daily
        fatigue), 148–49
    5 (total revitalization), 149
    6 (breathing freely), 150
    7 (exhaling the dirt, dust,
        and greasy grime),
        150–51

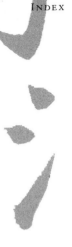

8 (inhaling the purified
breath of life), 151
fingers and toes, 145–59
    big toes and little fingers,
        157–59
    index fingers and ring toes,
        155–56
    index toes and ring fingers,
        157
    middle toes and middle
        fingers, 156–57
    thumbs and little toes,
        153–55
first aid, 161–69
first depth, 27, 29–31, 57
    safety energy locks of, 60–
        66
flows, 18, 41, 43–54, 96, 97
    defined, 44–45
    Diagonal Mediator, 52–54
    Main Central. *See* Main
        Central Flow
    Supervisor, 49–52, 54, 56, 96,
        98
    See also organ flows
fourth depth, 35–37, 57
    safety energy lock of, 90–92

Gall Bladder Function Energy,
    125–27
general daily sequences. *See*
    daily sequences

hands:
    feet linked with, 151–59
    as jumper cables, 23–25,
        27
    palms and soles: revitaliz-
        ing the entire being,
        152–53
    See also finger poses
        (mudras); fingers and
        toes
harmony, 18, 99–100
    See also disharmonies
        (labels)
Heart Function Energy,
    110–13

Jin Shin Jyutsu:
    as art, not technique, 24
    core concepts of, 18–19
    foundations of, 11–21
    frequently asked questions
        about, 171–73
    life energy balanced by,
        12–14; *See also* life
        energy
    meaning of name, 14, 16
jumper-cabling, 23–25, 27

Kidney Function Energy,
    118–20

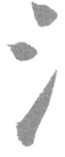

labels. *See* disharmonies (labels)

Large Intestine Function Energy, 103–6

life energy, 12–14, 18–19
    ascending, 46
    attitudes and, 18; *See also* attitudes
    blocked. *See* disharmonies
    breath as expression of, 18; *See also* breath
    depths of, 18; *See also* depths
    descending, 46
    flows of, 18, 44; *See also* flows
    hands as jumper cables for, 23–25
    oval movement of, 19, 45
    safety energy locks and, 19; *See also* safety energy locks (SELs)

Liver Function Energy, 128–30

Lung Function Energy, 101–3

Main Central Flow, 45–49, 54, 98
    Diagonal Mediator Flows and, 52
    palms and soles related to, 152–53

project for harmonizing, 46–48

Martin, Celeste, 1–3, 5–6

Meader, Pat, 2–3

Mediator Flows, 52
    project for harmonizing, 52–54

mudras. *See* finger poses (mudras)

Murai, Jiro, 4, 8, 14–17, 43, 44, 98, 145, 146, 151–52

ninth depth, 26

organ flows, 97–131
    biorhythms and, 100
    Bladder Function Energy, 115–17, 141
    circuit of, 98
    Diaphragm Function Energy, 120–22
    disharmonies and, 99–100
    Gall Bladder Function Energy, 125–27
    Heart Function Energy, 110–13
    Kidney Function Energy, 118–20

Large Intestine Function
Energy, 103–6
Liver Function Energy,
128–30
Lung Function Energy,
101–3
Small Intestine Function
Energy, 113–15
Spleen Function Energy, 99,
108–10, 135
Stomach Function Energy,
99, 106–8, 137
Umbilicus Function Energy,
122–24
organs, depths and, 27
diaphragm, umbilicus, 28
heart, small intestine, 38, 39
kidney, bladder, 36
liver, gall bladder, 34
lung, large intestine, 32
spleen, stomach, 30

posterior descending energy
sequence, 134, 141–42
pretense (cover-up), 18

sadness, 18
safety energy locks (SELs), 19,
55–80, 81–96, 100
1 (the prime mover), 60–61

2 (wisdom), 62
3 (the door), 63–64
4 (the window), 64–66
5 (regeneration), 66–67
6 (balance and
discrimination), 67–68
7 (victory), 68–70
8 (rhythm, strength, and
peace), 70–71
9 (ending of one cycle,
beginning of another),
71–73
10 (warehouse of
abundance), 73–74
11 (unloading the burdens
of the past and future),
74–75
12 (not my will but thy will),
75–76
13 (love your enemies),
76–77
14 (equilibrium, sustenance),
77–78
15 (wash our hearts with
laughter), 78–80
16 (transformation), 82–83
17 (reproductive energy),
83–84
18 (body consciousness and
personality), 84–85
19 (perfect balance), 85–86
20 (everlasting eternity),
86–87
21 (profound security and

escape from mental
bondage), 87–88
22 (complete adaptation),
88–90
23 (controller of human
destiny, proper
circulation maintenance),
90, 91–92
24 (harmonizing chaos),
92–94
25 (quietly regenerating),
94–95
26 (the director, total peace,
total harmony), 95
first-depth, 60–66
second-depth, 66–79
third-depth, 82–90
fourth-depth, 90–92
fifth-depth, 92–96
depths and, 56–57
index of, for particular
needs, 58
precision in locating, 58, 135
second depth, 32–33, 57
safety energy locks of, 66–79
seventh depth, 26
sixth depth, 28–29, 45, 57
Small Intestine Function
Energy, 113–15

Spleen Function Energy, 99,
108–10, 135
Stomach Function Energy, 99,
106–8, 137
Supervisor Flows, 49–52, 54,
56, 96, 98
Diagonal Mediator Flows
and, 52
project for, 50–51
symptoms. *See* conditions

third depth, 33–34, 57
safety energy locks of, 82–90
thirty-six breaths, 21
toes. *See* fingers and toes

Umbilicus Function Energy,
122–24

worry, 18

about the authors

Alice Burmeister attended her first Jin Shin Jyutsu seminar taught by Mary Burmeister in 1982. After studying with Mary Burmeister for several years she became a practitioner and has continued her involvement with the art ever since. Alice currently resides in Scottsdale, Arizona, with her husband, David, and their son, Matthew.

Tom Monte is the best-selling author of 17 books, including *The Complete Guide to Natural Healing, World Medicine, The Ten Best Tools to Boost Your Immune System* (with Elinor Levy, Ph.D.), *Natural Prozac* (with Joel Robertson, Ph.D.), and *Recalled by Life* (with Anthony Sattilaro, M.D.). He lives with his wife and three children in Amherst, Massachusetts.